Praise for *Unhooked*

"A riveting and shocking book. Laura Stepp's superb investigative work raises questions that are as compelling as they are appalling. Are young women accepting as okay sexual behavior that isn't okay and never has been? Can girls really act like boys and get away with it emotionally? What happens when boys who have no sexual boundaries placed upon them grow up to be men? This is a book you can't stop reading and you won't stop talking about." —Patricia Cornwell

"Stepp's arguments are rooted in rigorous firsthand reporting, as the book took her to the front lines of today's sexual battlefield. . . . She does a good job of differentiating between the 'free love' of her collegiate days (and the periods that followed it) and the situation as it currently exists." —*San Francisco Chronicle*

"Thought-provoking." —*The Washington Post*

"Stepp wisely allows the women's stories to speak for themselves." —*Washington City Paper*

"*Unhooked* is the title of [Stepp's] new book, but she doesn't mean it only in a physical sense. Hooking up also causes young women to be emotionally unhooked from a partner and from themselves." —*The Boston Globe*

"Stepp is a genius at getting adolescents, teenagers, and young adults to talk openly about their private lives. For parents who care about their children's welfare, Stepp's words are always educational—and almost always shocking." —*St. Louis Post-Dispatch*

"Eye-opening and powerful, Stepp's book also offers empowering advice for women as they navigate today's sexual landscape."

—*Kirkus Reviews*

"Every parent, college administrator, and student will benefit from this study of the hookup culture on college campuses across America. Stepp focuses her scholarly journalism on the most intimate sexual and emotional details of college life, explaining concepts such as 'battle buddy,' 'date auction,' and 'freakin',' and the result is an extraordinarily candid depiction and a set of remarkable findings. Although freedom for these girls has replaced intimacy, their emotional needs are poignantly described. This is a pathbreaking study—one not soon forgotten." —H. Keith H. Brodie, M.D.,
President-Emeritus, Duke University

"[Stepp's] book offers a rare combination of intelligence—on the part of the author, her subjects, and the experts' quotes—and insight regarding the sexual landscape of today's adolescents."

—*Library Journal*

"Alarming." —*St. Paul Pioneer Press*

"A compelling account of the causes and potential consequences of a noteworthy change in the sexual mores of contemporary American youth—the decoupling of physical and emotional intimacy. Laura Stepp weaves together case studies, hard data, and expert opinion in a narrative that is engaging and forceful without resorting to exaggeration. It's an important and provocative book."

—Laurence Steinberg, Ph.D., Temple University,
coauthor of *You and Your Adolescent: A Parent's Guide for Ages 10–20*, and author of *The 10 Basic Principles of Good Parenting*

"Young people talk candidly to Laura Stepp about their sexual and social lives because she listens with an open mind and a generous heart. Their stories provide hard but essential truths. *Unhooked* is on my must-read list for parents and their high school– and college-age children."
— Deborah Roffman, human sexuality educator
and author of *Sex and Sensibility*

"A remarkable book: astute, insightful, and rigorously reported. It demands the attention of all of us."
—William Raspberry, Duke University professor,
columnist, and author of *Looking Backward at Us*

"In this book, Stepp has lifted the veil of secrecy around young people and sex, and revealed the good, the bad, and the downright ugly."
—Sarah S. Brown, Executive Director,
National Campaign to Prevent Teen
and Unplanned Pregnancy

"In *Unhooked*, Laura Stepp contributes insight as illuminating as Betty Friedan's in *The Feminine Mystique*. Her astute analysis and stories will change how we educate and counsel young women."
—Judith Steinhart, Ed.D., co-creator
of the Go Ask Alice! website and coauthor
of *The "Go Ask Alice" Book of Answers*

"Anyone who's thought they might be losing the 'hookup' game should read this book. As should any single woman under thirty-five. As should parents."
—*Austin American-Statesman*

Also by Laura Sessions Stepp

Our Last Best Shot: Guiding Our Children

Through Early Adolescence

How Young Women

Pursue Sex,

Delay Love

and Lose at Both

unhooked

Laura Sessions Stepp

RIVERHEAD BOOKS

New York

RIVERHEAD BOOKS
Published by the Penguin Group
Penguin Group (USA) Inc.
375 Hudson Street, New York, New York 10014, USA
Penguin Group (Canada), 90 Eglinton Avenue East, Suite 700, Toronto, Ontario M4P 2Y3, Canada (a
division of Pearson Penguin Canada Inc.) • Penguin Books Ltd., 80 Strand, London WC2R
0RL, England • Penguin Group Ireland, 25 St. Stephen's Green, Dublin 2, Ireland (a division of
Penguin Books Ltd.) • Penguin Group (Australia), 250 Camberwell Road, Camberwell, Victoria 3124,
Australia (a division of Pearson Australia Group Pty. Ltd.) • Penguin Books India Pvt. Ltd., 11
Community Centre, Panchsheel Park, New Delhi–110 017, India • Penguin Group (NZ), 67 Apollo
Drive, Rosedale, North Shore 0632, New Zealand (a division of Pearson New Zealand Ltd.) • Penguin
Books (South Africa) (Pty.) Ltd., 24 Sturdee Avenue, Rosebank, Johannesburg 2196, South Africa

Penguin Books Ltd., Registered Offices: 80 Strand, London WC2R 0RL, England

The publisher has no control over and does not assume any responsibility for author or
third-party websites or their content.

Throughout this book, the names of some individuals and their personal details have been changed.

Excerpt from "Bring 'Em Out": words and music by Kenneth Gamble, Thom Bell, Roland Lawrence
Chambers, Clifford Harris, Shawn Carter, and Kasseem Dean © 2004 Warner-Tamerlane Publishing
Corp., WB Music Corp. and Domani and Ya Majesty's Music. All rights on behalf of itself and Domani
and Ya Majesty's Music administered by WB Music Corp. All rights reserved. Used by permission of Alfred
Publishing Co., Inc.
Excerpts from *The Chronicle* © 2004 Duke University. Used by permission of *The Chronicle*.
Excerpt from "This Much I Do Remember" from *Picnic, Lightning* by Billy Collins © 1998. Reprinted
by permission of the University of Pittsburgh Press.

First Riverhead hardcover edition: February 2007
First Riverhead trade paperback edition: February 2008
Riverhead trade paperback ISBN: 978-1-59448-284-7

The Library of Congress has catalogued the Riverhead hardcover edition as follows:

Stepp, Laura Sessions.
Unhooked : how young women pursue sex, delay love and lose at both / Laura Sessions Stepp.
p.   cm.
ISBN 978-1-59448-938-9
1. Man-woman relationships—United States.   2. Girls—Sexual behavior—United States.
3. Dating (Social customs)—United States.   4. Women college students—United States—
Social life and customs.   I. Title.
HQ801.S82   2007   2006037171
306.73084'220973—dc22

PRINTED IN THE UNITED STATES OF AMERICA
10 9 8 7 6 5 4 3 2 1

For Carl

Contents

Foreword

BY ALICIA

I f there's one thing I know about adults, it's that they pounce on the subject of adolescent sexuality with zeal. Teachers, doctors, psychologists, parents and talk-show hosts express both distaste and concern for my generation's in-your-face, supersize-me, consumer attitude toward sex. Yet in all that we've read and heard, when have we gotten an insider's perspective?

Adults look at the sex lives of children through a lens ground in the past. This limits their ability to capture and understand the world today. In this book, Laura Stepp doesn't do this. Instead, she has taken time to observe and listen as other young women and I struggled to develop our ideas about sex and love: how both should be given and received, and what we deserve from each. She has looked through *our* lenses and attempted to synthesize *our* perspectives. Ever the journalist, she has worked hard to get the inside scoop.

. . .

Walking toward the bus stop on a mild fall day in Durham, North Carolina, I wasn't sure I'd recognize her. She had interviewed me several years before for an article in *The Washington Post,* but our communication since had been limited. I was excited, however, by our reunion because I remembered fondly the mutual intellectual respect I'd felt in our first conversations. I scanned the faces of college students milling about until I spotted the dainty figure of a woman about my mother's age.

She was neatly dressed à la Ann Taylor, poised and gentle in mannerism and appearance and hardly the person you'd think would request an interview about "hooking up," the intentionally vague term my generation uses to represent any possible amalgam of sexual behaviors.

I was twenty and a junior at Duke University, tackling the core of my engineering major. I had come to college knowing I had a lot to figure out about myself, no small part of which involved relationships. Laura wanted to observe me over the course of the school year. She asked me to talk to her about the hookup culture: what it was, the extent to which I participated, and what I thought about it. Looking at me over the rims of her glasses, smile lines crinkling just around her eyes, she asked me to define "hooking up." No, really, like, she wanted to know: Was it sex or blow jobs or what?

That first interview started our two-year collaboration, a friendship marked off in salads, coffee and sinful desserts, and measured in conversations, recorded in Laura's spidery mom-cursive sprawling across the pages of whatever miniature notebook she happened to have with her at the time. Her questions seemed simple enough at first, but as she probed, I discovered the answers weren't simple. I also realized that hooking up had influenced my notions of self-worth, love, relationships and expectations of men in ways I hadn't realized.

She was a cool observer, happy to spend a night out at local pubs and clubs, asking countless questions about what was going on and why. She was not writing an exposé to criticize and demean young women, but she *was* asking questions that were always personal, and sometimes painful and embarrassing. She left no issue unaddressed, forcing me to think about what I had accepted unquestioningly as the norm. I knew it would be a startling thing to see my personal sexual escapades in print, but I trusted Laura and her motivations.

I've invested my time and thought in *Unhooked* because I believe in it. I've grown up through these conversations, and Laura and I have learned from each other. We don't agree all the time, but there's something to be said for simply talking. Our discussions have helped me define love for myself, and in doing so I've gained an appreciation for how important a process that is.

You don't need to agree with all the perspectives in this book, nor relate to all the stories young women have contributed. *Unhooked* is simply a starting point for discussion, a strong argument for the importance of talking about relationships, period.

To my peers I'd like to say: Our generation is wonderfully outspoken, but it's time we learned to listen as well. Who we love is a reflection of what we value, so what do we value? We would do well to examine our lives and the roles that love and sex play in them. This book will catalyze such introspection.

And to parents: One thing I've come to appreciate post-adolescence is that you're eager to give us the very best. One critical way to do that is to engage more fully in our lives. Listen not only to Laura but to us, your children, as we transition from child to adult. Address our sexuality in a truly interactive conversation. Take a lesson from the open-minded, genuine, no-holds-barred attitude with which Laura approached the subject of *Unhooked*.

Our society is obsessed with sex, but no one wants to talk frankly about sex. Even now, I'm writing under a pseudonym, not because I'm ashamed of what I've done, but because I need protection from the stigma society places on those who publicize the messy details of their skirmishes with sex and love. If I could sign my name to this foreword without fear of losing my job or getting slandered in the media down the road, I would. I'm proud of how I've learned from my failures as well as my successes. I suspect the other young women in this book feel the same way.

Regardless of whose story you're reading, what is being said is important. Silence perpetuates stigmas, and stigmas prevent understanding.

So let's talk about sex, baby.

Introduction

I can explain the origin of this book with two stories—one brief, the other more detailed.

In the spring of 1998, the principal of a suburban Washington, D.C., middle school called about twenty-five parents to a special night meeting. There, over the annoying hum of the fluorescent bulbs found in eighth-grade classrooms around the country, she announced that as many as a dozen girls had been performing oral sex on two or three boys for most of the school year. The thirteen- and fourteen-year-old students were getting it on at parties, in parks and even in a couple of neighborhood parking lots.

The parents sat momentarily in silence, stunned. This was before President Bill Clinton and Monica Lewinsky made oral sex a household word, and two years before the popularity of oral sex in middle schools percolated through the media. One mother, who had heard the news over the phone from a school counselor before the meeting, told me later, "I almost dropped the phone."

The school was my son's. He was not involved, but kids he knew were. I wrote about the sex ring for *The Washington Post* and I remember, to this day, what one girl in particular told me.

"I did it first in the fall with a boy I kinda liked, thinking it would make him like me," she said. "It didn't. Then I did it a couple more times in the spring at parties. We would go outside, then come back in and sit around and talk about it. It was no big deal."

Now, in 1964, my eighth-grade girlfriends and I were no prisses; we had secret places around town where we went to kiss and neck with our boyfriends. But when did teenaged girls—everyday girls, not just the "fast" girls or the "loose" girls—start skipping the smooching and go straight to giving head? How did they come to believe that offering their services to guys they barely knew "was no big deal"?

My reporting instincts shifted into high gear as I discovered that this was not an isolated case. School administrators were beginning to report similar behaviors in middle schools around the Washington area. My editors, extremely uncomfortable about putting the phrases "oral sex" and "middle school" in the same newspaper story, pressed for multiple, concrete examples, and I delivered. Eventually, after much debate, they published the article on the front page, and that launched me on an investigation that continues today into the sexual and romantic lives of America's young people.

Now for the second, longer story. It took place almost seven years later, in January 2005, on a college campus in downtown Washington.

Rapper T.I.'s voice—and more than a few shots of liquor—had hundreds of students buzzed that Saturday night inside the Marvin Center of George Washington University (or GW). Crowded along both sides of an elevated catwalk, waiting for scantily clad freshman women to emerge from a tent at one end, the students sang along with the music:

Who set the city on fire as soon as he got freed
Da king back now, ho's don't even know how to act now
Hit the club strippers gettin' naked 'fore I sit down
Bring 'em out! Bring 'em out!

Out they came, one act after another, eighteen- and nineteen-year-old Division I athletes, ranging from passably pretty to drop-dead gorgeous, putting themselves up for bid at the annual "date auction" sponsored by GW's student athletic council. Big white bidding cards popped up immediately. Fifty dollars for a night on the town with a couple of lacrosse players! Seventy-five dollars for members of the crew team!

The water polo players, dressed in swim parkas and strappy black stilettos, brought down the house. They had been practicing polo for eight months, spending thirty hours a week in the pool. Their season over, they left little question in anyone's mind that they were ready to party.

Bumping and grinding to a new rap number, they ripped off their jackets to reveal short nightgowns—see-through black, with pink polka dots—over black bras and lacy fuchsia boy shorts.

Fifty dollars! The bidding began.

A couple of players started to strip further and, drunk out of their minds, fell down.

Seventy-five dollars!

One player pretended to go down on another girl.

Eighty dollars!

Morgan, a muscular blonde freshman, started flashing the audience.

One hundred dollars! Sold!

Morgan turned to wobble back boozily into the tent.

"Nice vagina!" yelled a boy standing just below her as she left.

The next thing Morgan knew, it was early morning and she was lying in her own bed next to someone she thought of as just a friend. He told her that they had hooked up after the auction and that she had been a willing partner.

He also told her that they had had sex. After inspecting herself briefly, she realized it was true.

Four months later, she sat across a table from me in a campus coffee shop, her hair pulled back by a Burberry plaid headband. She sketched out the rest of that year at college. She'd had a series of sexual encounters, and none of them amounted to anything. She depended on alcohol to get ready for boys and, when things didn't work out, to take the edge off her disappointment. Her grades were falling, putting her at risk of losing her scholarship. She had had several sessions with a psychiatrist, who prescribed an antidepressant that made her groggy.

"I've dug myself a pretty deep ditch," she admitted.

Would she participate in a date auction again, knowing what she knew now? I asked.

"Absolutely," she said. "It was so much fun. The energy, the hype . . . The next day everyone was saying, 'Those water polo girls were outrageous.' . . . I knew I was an object, yeah. But I didn't feel like a piece of meat at all. If it was in any way degrading, I never would've done it."

Listening to her in the spring of 2005, my mind went back to 1968 again and I found myself making generational comparisons once more. Sure, we used to leave our college dorm windows cracked so our boyfriends could sneak in. But we were terrified of being found out and wouldn't think of taking off our clothes until the guys were inside and the lights were off. Now girls were stripping in the student center in front of dozens of boys they didn't know, pantomiming sex onstage and later doing the real thing without saying much, if anything, to their partners. When did conversation and negotiation drop completely out of the picture?

Clearly, young women have changed not only the way they relate intimately to young men but also the way they think about intimacy. My *Post* articles on sexuality since the oral-sex scandal have not been about isolated acts of a promiscuous few but indications of a large cultural shift. To some degree, depending on their temperament, upbringing and luck, all girls are caught up in the changes. Young people have virtually abandoned dating and replaced it with group get-togethers and sexual behaviors that are detached from love or commitment—and sometimes even from liking. High school and college teachers I've talked to, as well as researchers, remark on this. Relationships have been replaced by the casual sexual encounters known as hookups. Love, while desired by some, is being put on hold or seen as impossible; sex is becoming the primary currency of social interaction. Some girls can handle this; others, like Morgan, are exhausted physically, emotionally and spiritually by it. They struggle largely outside the awareness of parents who either don't know what is going on or are vaguely aware but don't know what to do.

Science tells us that sexual attractiveness plays a significant role in the emotional and social lives of young women. Parents seem largely unaware of this or of how firmly hooking up has taken hold in young people's imaginations and lives. They are reassured by statistics that show a significant decline in teen pregnancies and a slight drop in the proportion of high school students having intercourse. What they don't understand is that sexual intercourse, or any other sexual act, is only part of the story. What is—or isn't—going on *in addition to* sex is at least as important.

The crucial thing to remember in all of this is that hooking up, in the minds of this generation, carries no commitment. Partners hook up with the understanding that however far they go sexually, neither should become romantically involved in any serious way. Hooking up's defining characteristic is the ability to *unhook* from a partner at any time, just as they might delete an old song on their iPod or an out-of-date "away" message on their computer. Maybe they tire of their partner, or find someone who is "hotter" or, for some other reason, more to their liking. Maybe they get burned badly in a relationship, or find themselves swamped with term papers and final exams. The freedom to unhook from someone—ostensibly without repercussions—gives them maximum flexibility. Although I use both phrases, this is not a hookup culture so much as an unhooked culture. It is a way of thinking about relationships, period.

One can see this same impermanence in some of their other commitments—to their jobs and their life plans, for example. In their personal lives, many young women carry it with them as they move through their twenties, when the "hookup buddy" becomes the "sometime boyfriend." One national study found that among eighteen- to twenty-nine-year-olds, only slightly more than a third were in committed relationships. Of the rest, more said they were not looking than looking.

This book explores, through the eyes of real girls and young women, how complex this unhooked culture is, how firmly entrenched and how it has affected the thoughts, feelings, behaviors and aspirations of this generation—including those girls who want no part of it. Of particular interest to me, having come of age during the women's movement of the late 1960s and early 1970s, is that the new sexual landscape has been designed in part by girls, to the delight of guys who no longer have to work very hard for girls' attention or their bodies. Young women's goal was, at one time, to save their bodies and their reputations for someone they loved, while young men were encouraged to play the field. Young men are still expected to be players, but now young women have jumped into the arena with them. And so I have chosen to focus my attention on these female architects. How do they feel about their new freedom? Great or used? Loved or lonely? Free or trapped in unexpected ways? What do they really think about relationships, including marriage?

Shortly before I started my research, I spent three hours talking to four young working-class women in their early twenties about men and sex. Never once during the conversation did they use the word "love." When I finally pointed this out, one of them explained, "Sex is different from love." The other three nodded.

On another morning I watched a half-dozen girls who had just graduated from an exclusive Virginia high school padding around a North Carolina beach house in camisole tops and low-slung pajama bottoms, cooking breakfast for guy friends and listening to music that would make their mothers blush. It occurred to me that these young women did not worry, as their mothers did, about showing off their imperfect bodies. They did not shy away from talking frankly about sex. As they move through college and into jobs, they might be less apt to worry, as their mothers did, about compromising their identity or independence in bed. These were good things.

But who, I wondered, was telling them that they were worth taking more care with—that they deserved to take care with themselves and insist that boys take care with them, too? Who was reminding them that sex, in any form, is more powerful when you don't throw it around, more satisfying when it's savored with someone you love? Who was asking them to think seriously about their goals for happiness beyond the law degree or to consider that having sex with lots of men might limit their ability to sustain a long-term commitment as well as their ability to conceive children? Who was helping them see that loving relationships are uniquely satisfying and manageable—and need not tie them down for the rest of their lives?

As I explained my research to acquaintances in my neighborhood, church and job, I would often hear something along the lines of "What is wrong with these girls?" That is not the right question. The question should be how this came to be, and what, if anything, should be done about it. Loving may be as basic as breathing, but loving well is a learned behavior. Who and where are young women's teachers?

. . .

The research was a natural outgrowth of my previous book, *Our Last Best Shot*. In that book, I wrote about ten- to fifteen-year-olds who, as young adolescents, were beginning to shape a self-image based in part on whether they felt loved and capable of love. The romantic encounters the younger ones, boys as well as girls, enjoyed were short-lived and confined to passing notes, messaging each other on the computer and stealing kisses at school dances when no one was looking. But starting in eighth grade, things changed: Kids thought nothing of sneaking to movies with a boyfriend or girlfriend or going to parties where couples made out. Girls were as likely to pursue as be pursued, and the pressure to "go all the way" (the old-fashioned expression used by two ninth-grade girls I interviewed in a small Kansas town) was intermittent but occasionally intense.

In general, however, the struggles these younger adolescents had with boyfriends and girlfriends were of less importance than the battles they waged with parents and peers. That tends to be true with most teens until the later years of high school and particularly in college, when adolescents begin to focus seriously on the kind of romantic partners they are becoming. What does that exploration look like? I wondered as I prepared to start this book.

I began with scientific reports, and didn't find much that was helpful. Sex research, sorely underfunded in this country, has been confined primarily to younger teenagers, and survey questions are worded in a way that rarely matches the language that teenagers use, leaving one wondering how well the findings match what teens are really doing. Nonetheless, I commissioned my own analysis of available data and am grateful to the independent organization Child Trends for help in making sense of the most reliable large-scale studies.

We found, for example, that the proportion of young women ages eighteen to twenty-two who reported having intercourse—seventy-five percent—equaled that of young men. Seventy percent of both sexes had had sex before their nineteenth birthdays. Only one-third of young women said they truly wanted to have sex the first time they did so, compared to one-half of the young men. One particularly interesting finding was that while two out of three young men said it was better to get married than go through life single, fewer than half of the young women felt that way.

Statistics do not talk, however, they only point us to the people to whom we need to talk. The heart of the book, then, became the insights provided by the most important people: Alicia, Sienna and the other young women whose personal lives fill the following chapters.

The need to be connected intimately to others is as central to our well-being as food and shelter. In my view, if we don't get it right, we're probably not going to get anything else in life right. My goal for this book stems from this premise and is twofold. First, I hope to encourage girls to think hard about whether they're "getting it right," whether their sexual and romantic experiences are contributing to—or destroying—their sense of self-worth and strength. Their studied effort to remain uncommitted convinces me only of how strongly they want to be attached.

Second, I hope to encourage adults, men as well as women, to have the kind of conversations with girls that I've had. If you're a woman reading this, put yourself in the shoes of the young woman you're reading about and ask what you would have done in her situation. As a man, think of these girls as your daughters and ask yourself what you hope your daughter would do. You may want to separate yourself from these women—I know I did—but you end up realizing you can't, because they and their partners are wrestling with the same needs and desires we all share at some level.

Discussion over a period of time can help girls make wiser choices; I've seen it happen. One college junior, on the heels of a rough period with a guy she was hooking up with, talked to me at lunch one day for a couple of hours. Several days later, I received an upbeat e-mail. "Conversation with adults is a big part of why I've begun to feel better about myself," she wrote. "Really my happiest moment at home during those two weeks was our conversation that Tuesday."

Such conversation takes place only if we approach young people hoping to understand rather than intending to censure. This book is written to further that effort by showing grayheads what the current sexual culture, so different from the one we remember, is like. The book is full of terms that will be new, even shocking, to some readers. We don't have to adopt these terms—just as we need not agree with everything young people do—but we do need to know what the terms and actions mean and don't mean to those involved.

Many adults, protective in other parts of their children's lives, turn a blind eye to sexual matters. How else to explain Lingerie Barbie dolls purchased for three- and four-year-olds? Or parents spending a hundred dollars at Club Libby Lu so their kindergarteners can dress up in spandex and sparkles and learn how to shimmy and shake it on a catwalk? By the time they're in middle school, girls are reading young-adult novels such as *Rainbow Party*, in which a high school sophomore invites her girlfriends to perform oral sex on a group of boys. By high school, girls and guys can watch videotapes of themselves having sex or, with the help of a webcam, their friends having sex.

"In many of these situations," says Deborah Roffman, a teacher who lectures nationally about sex education, "it is clear that adults are complicit, either by their neglect, cluelessness or even subtle encouragement."

Although familiar with Roffman and the efforts of organizations such as the National Campaign to Prevent Teen Pregnancy, I had not realized the depth of adults' reluctance to talk openly about sex among teenagers until I wrote a story for the *Post* about girls keeping track of how many guys they had hooked up with.

These young women chatted about their numbers as if they were compiling data in a brokerage firm. They kept count in planners stowed away in bedside tables and typed names on Excel spreadsheets along with details and grades for performance. One of them, a college senior, described in my story how common this practice had been at her Catholic high school, which I did not name.

She later regretted being so honest. Early on the morning that she was to take a summer job in the development office of her college, which was also Catholic, an administrator called to rescind the job offer, citing her quotes in the newspaper. That same day, her parents told her to stop talking to me. I heard also from a friend whose daughter attended that particular Catholic high school and had helped me on other stories. My friend informed me coolly that her daughter was to have no more contact with me ever, on any story.

How, I wondered at the time, can we expect young people to make good decisions about their sexuality—the essence of what it means to be female or male—when adults they know resist discussing it publicly and thereby deny its central place in all of our lives?

To observe this culture in depth, I interviewed dozens of young women, ages sixteen to twenty-one and white, black, Latin, Asian and Middle Eastern. These girls had grown up in various communities across the country and attended public and private schools and universities on the East Coast. Slightly more than half of them had been raised by two biological parents. They shared one significant demographic: Their families were at least moderately well-off. This meant that regardless of race, ethnicity or the address they called home, they dressed similarly, shared the same jargon, listened and danced to the same music, used the same technology to communicate and related to their friends and families in similar ways.

I decided early to focus mainly on women enrolled in four-year colleges for several reasons. The majority of high school graduates now start at such a college or university, although some don't finish. I could talk freely with college women, who are legal adults. I also would have more freedom to follow them throughout their days and nights as they went about their various activities with various friends and in various moods. College women also appealed because it is in college where young women first begin to contemplate seriously the traits they want in a life partner—and to my surprise, when I began my investigating, I found that little had been written about that struggle in popular nonfiction.

Much of my work at the *Post* had centered on middle school and high school students, and I knew that decisions in late adolescence are based partly on experiences during these earlier "gateway" years. So I decided to begin the book with high school girls.

The reader will notice that I use the words "girl" and "girls" in this book, along with "young woman" and "young women." That is because female college students, and even some women in their twenties and thirties, call themselves girls. This practice puzzles those of us who came of age during the women's movement and demanded that we be called women as soon as we reached eighteen, just as boys became men at that age. But it reflects, I think, the way young women, particularly those in middle- and upper-income families, have been protected, even coddled, to the point where they think of themselves as not yet adults. Economics and social custom play a part in this. Adulthood, in the conventional sense, means getting a job, leaving home and starting a family. As young women, like young men, postpone these milestones, they remain stuck being not quite adolescents but also not quite adults.

I have changed the names of the girls, using names they chose for themselves, and left out some of the details of their lives. I also changed the names of their family members, friends and partners.

I chose subjects who: illustrated something surprising or significant about the hookup culture; could articulate clearly what was happening to them and their friends in this culture; and seemed candid but not prone to exaggeration. Because of the sensitive nature of the information they would be sharing, it was important to have easy, personal access to them. I did not want to be confined to e-mails and telephone calls as means of discussing blow jobs and date rape. Ultimately, I selected three girls in Washington, D.C.–area high schools, two public and one private, and six young women at two universities I could get to quickly: George Washington University, in D.C., and Duke University, a four-hour drive away in Durham, North Carolina. At Duke, campus social life was driven largely by thirty-eight fraternities and sororities. This was not so at George Washington, with twenty Greek organizations and a much larger student body. Officials at both universities were open and cooperative, and I should add that the observations I make about these two institutions could be made about many other schools.

I taught a course on love, sexuality and the media in George Washington's School of Media and Public Affairs, and those students contributed enormously to my understanding. I also observed and corresponded with two girls who identified themselves as lesbians—one at Brown University in Providence, Rhode Island, and the other at the tiny University of Mary Washington in Fredericksburg, Virginia. At year's end, after extensive discussion with one of those girls, I decided to include neither in the book because I believed they were distinct in many ways. It is not that they didn't hook up or relate to their partners in some of the same ways as the straight girls. But they also had other issues—of identity and disclosure, for example—that complicated their stories and made them unique. And their power struggles were with other girls, not with guys.

I came to this decision reluctantly. The gay female population is larger than we used to think. According to a recent national study, 8 percent of high school girls report having had some kind of sexual experience with another girl. For older girls, that figure increases to 14 percent. Americans frequently assume that young women all speak in the same voice, when they most certainly do not. Gay and bisexual girls need to have a separate account written of their hookup world, and I hope someone will do that.

I spent time in class with the girls in this book, attended sporting events and plays, and sat with them in coffee shops and restaurants. I shopped with them (improving my wardrobe considerably) and partied with them. Some of the most memorable moments were observed from a bar stool—a scene I hadn't been a part of in more years than I care to admit. Occasionally, on returning to my hotel at, say, two a.m., I would call my husband and say, "I am way too old to be doing this." But I also enjoyed being with them, and now, frankly, I miss them and their energy, enthusiasm and challenge to my ideas.

I interviewed the friends and boyfriends of these girls, visited the girls in their homes and talked to some of their parents. I listened with interest as mothers and fathers told me how little they knew about their daughters' sexual and romantic lives. I was intrigued that some seemed not particularly concerned about that. Parental anxieties were reserved for grades and plans for graduate school and careers—a reality that, as you will see in later chapters, has important repercussions for girls' private lives.

What will you read in this book, and through whose story? In Section One, you will read first about the hooking-up phenomenon itself—its definition, scope and short history—through the story of a Duke senior I called Jamie. I chose Jamie in part because she hooked up during her first year at Duke and then moved into a deeper, more lasting relationship that gave her some perspective on her earlier experiences. You will see how hooking up can blindside an unsuspecting freshman; how it has become not just a temporary fancy but a replacement for dating, affecting even those who, against the odds, date; and how young women, empowered by Title IX–inspired success in school and on the playing field, have been the driving force behind this change.

Whether they're looking to hook up serially or, less often, for something more substantial, what young women want most is control over the guys they've set out to conquer. In Section Two, through the stories of Sienna, Anna and Mieka, you'll see what the contest looks like in high school and the influence that friends have in egging each other on. You'll also witness the kind of influence parents have on girls' choices. Sienna and Anna were close to their mothers; Mieka was close to neither parent.

Section Two ends with Nicole, a George Washington sophomore, who illustrates that, while hooking up may seem like a game in high school, it becomes a serious campaign in college, the prize being the ability to walk away at will. Nicole's experience suggests that as a result of hooking up, close friendships between girls have replaced long-term relationships with guys. Without parents or college authorities helping them figure out how to navigate the new social terrain, college women depend on their gal pals to push them out there and then protect them from going too far.

Nicole was a closet romantic. Indeed, most of the girls I observed came across initially as ball-busters, but privately, either late at night or after a couple of drinks, they morphed into softer versions of Bridget Jones, hoping for someone to knock on their door, flowers in hand. As hard as they tried to run away from love, they ended up falling in love, usually only briefly, and were reluctant to call it anything but "having feelings for."

So why did they continue to hook up? Section Three, which shares the stories of Shaida, Cleo and Victoria, suggests three reasons: the ethic of female empowerment; parental expectations for academic and professional achievement; and reluctance on the part of authorities on campus to intervene in students' social lives.

Shaida was a declared feminist who arrived at college assuming, as many older feminists do, that girls who feel powerful in the classroom will act in their own best interests in the bedroom. Personal and painful experiences changed her mind—and also made her believe that feminism needs to revisit its assumptions and expand its vision of what it means to be a woman.

Cleo was Nicole's older sister. Their mother was a successful lawyer who wanted her daughters to prepare themselves for a successful life with or without husbands. Cleo, internalizing her mother's and father's hopes, grew up believing that she should ace the SATs and later the foreign service exam, star on a winning basketball team, date someone equally talented, graduate from college summa cum laude and move on to a top graduate school, all without breaking a sweat. She fell in love her junior year in college but, unable to see how the relationship could work in the perfect future she envisioned for herself, also hooked up on the side. Interestingly, although both sisters were influenced by their parents' dreams, and both attended the same university, Cleo, more than Nicole, ended up confused and uncertain—the result, in part, of their different temperaments.

In all these stories, the reader may be struck, as I was, by the total freedom that college students enjoy on campus today. They move from their years at home, when so many decisions are made for them, to a place where everything is up to them. College authorities, at one time surrogate parents, have become absentee landlords. Rules that both inhibited and protected students are gone. Although the pendulum is beginning to swing back in the direction of college control, the movement is slight, and Victoria's story shows how one young woman managed that freedom and at what cost. The religious rituals and beliefs that she brought from home helped ground her, as did a couple of college programs. Her parents' relationship, unlike that of some of the other parents in this book, provided a model for her of what she'd like to have one day in her own life. Early in the year, she decided that the only way to win at the hookup game was not to play, and these supports helped her maintain her resolve.

The early-twentieth-century British actress Beatrice Tanner Campbell, when asked about two actors who took an unusual liking to each other, reportedly replied, "Does it really matter what these affectionate people do, so long as they don't do it in the street and frighten the horses?" It is tempting to say the same thing about young women once they get to college. Section Four suggests why we shouldn't. As Alicia, a junior at Duke, helps us understand, hooking up regularly puts girls at risk both physically and emotionally. It also carries potential implications for their future roles as mothers, workers and members of a community.

Alicia came to college looking and feeling like the odd girl out, and she used hooking up to reassure herself that someone, or in her case, a series of someones, found her desirable despite her differences. This had consequences for her that, fortunately, because of her extraordinary observational powers, she was able to recognize and rectify.

One of my *Post* colleagues, reviewing a Katie Roiphe book, wrote that sex is not "the sum total of two people, a bed and a viral scare." How true. Sex in fact is a Rorschach test for how we treat all people—casually or with care. Skin to skin, we are at our most vulnerable, and so is our partner. We learn to trust or distrust, to give and receive in the most basic way possible, and we take those lessons with us into the wider world.

In that spirit, I end the book with "A Letter to Mothers and Daugh-

ters," a template for conversations we should be having with the next generation. These are not our daughters in the following pages. But they and
so many young women like them are the ones who will be teaching, doc-
toring and in other ways attending to our children and grandchildren.
Right now, they are trying to make sense of what is arguably the most
confusing sexual landscape any generation has ever faced.

Hooking Up: What It Means

JAMIE'S STORY

"The girls made all the effort.
The guys didn't have to do anything."
—JAMIE, TWENTY

Stroll across Duke University's East Campus late at night on any fall weekend, and you'll see them at the bus stop: clusters of young women sitting on concrete benches, pulling their thin, cropped cardigans tight against the wind that whips down the freshman yard of one of America's most prestigious universities. One girl rummages through her Fendi handbag. Another taps her Bebe heels impatiently on the pavement. Several of them check their watches as they wait for the blue-and-white bus that will take them on a twenty-minute ride to the Gothic dorms of West Campus, and the upperclassmen who have promised them a good time and all the Bud Light they can drink.

Jamie, a senior, knows this scene well. Three years ago, she was part of it. She was the one who went to the room of a guy she barely knew because it felt good to lie beside him, skin to skin, her head on his shoulder. She was the one who, at dawn, crawled out of the bed of a guy who didn't know her name because she woke up, saw he wasn't there and heard a girl in another room scream, "So, did you fuck her?"

She was the one who spent much of her first semester taking the bus from East to West to have sex with a senior named Jake and returning to East alone the next morning, even after he told her his feelings for her had cooled.

Back then, she wouldn't have called it hooking up, but that's what she calls it now.

I met Jamie immediately after a guest lecture at Duke in the early fall of 2004. My host, a professor who teaches a course on the family, had asked me to lead a class on hooking up. I anticipated a lively, intelligent discussion and was not disappointed. Duke students, drawn from around the country and abroad, are among America's most gifted. They score, on average, higher than 700 out of a possible 800 on the math and verbal portions of the traditional SATs, the standardized test universities use to select students. As Division I athletes, they are consistently ranked at or near the top nationally in basketball, tennis, soccer, cross-country and golf.

I was just starting my journey into the hookup culture. Prior to my visit to Duke, I had written several articles about hooking up for my newspaper, but more as an occasional tourist than a serious sojourner. I knew enough to know that I no longer needed just a road map; I needed a Michelin guide. Tom Wolfe's novel about sex at Duke had not yet been published, and the lacrosse sex scandal that roiled the campus and would attract national attention had not yet happened. I went to Duke because I had lectured on the campus in past years about other subjects and suspected that a new class might be able to provide me with some serious resources as I set out on my expedition.

They were a clean-cut bunch that afternoon, these twenty-five students sitting on carpeted tiers in front of me, and a far cry from the unshaven, slouching, somewhat morose classmates I remembered from my college years. Generational experts say their demographic group is more team-oriented, achievement-driven and polite than those of us who went to college in the late 1960s and 1970s. In appearance at least, that seemed to be the case. The young men, more than half of the class, wore khaki shorts, polo shirts and sandals, or designer jeans, supersized T-shirts and tennis shoes so clean they could have been purchased that day. The young women, in brightly colored skirts or neatly pressed shorts, were equally tailored. The classroom could have been a setting for late-1950s television except for two things—there were as many black students as whites, and we were talking about sex in a way that would have yanked any show off the air.

I first asked them to give me their definitions of hooking up.

"A physical encounter of affection," one smart aleck suggested, eliciting laughs from around the room.

"Third base and beyond," said another, followed quickly by, "More than making out," "Don't have to work at it," "Immediate gratification" and "Fast food."

I pushed them for additional descriptions and the tenor of their responses shifted: "No relationship," "Lack of communication," "Increases cynicism," "No emotional fulfillment," "Doesn't teach intimacy" and "Postpones marriage."

And "Easy to talk about."

So it was. The students described a work-hard, play-hard atmosphere at Duke that characterizes many elite colleges and universities. One-third of Duke's undergraduate men belonged to fraternities; one-half of the women were sorority members. Because Greek organizations' parties were open to anyone, the Greeks essentially were campus social life. Parties were one place hookups were arranged, the students said. But it also wasn't uncommon for a guy or girl to decide to take a study break and text-message a friend on a cell phone saying, "Let's roll." The students didn't seem particularly thrilled by the concept of hooking up, but it was clear that many had adopted it as a life form, for the present.

"If a girl offers, I'm not going to turn her down," said one guy whose frame was so tall it barely fit into his chair. "But I'm also not going to call her up and ask her for a date afterward."

This gave the professor the opportunity to jump in and attempt to make a case for "courtship"—a word that elicited a large amount of eyeball-rolling. Dating, he argued, encourages partners to put their best selves forward. A woman has more power when she holds her sexuality in reserve rather than play it out, he argued. A man who must prove his interest by asking a woman out to dinner is more likely to find that he is truly interested.

A cute, curly-haired female student raised her hand gingerly and I wondered for a split second whether she was going to agree with what seemed a convincing strategic argument. She didn't.

"That sounds like playing games," she said. "I don't have time to play games."

I decided to shift the conversation. How many of them wanted someday to be married? Virtually all hands went up.

The professor picked up on this. "Tell me, then, how do you go from hooking up to wedding vows?" Not a hand went up. Before he could continue, the bell rang and all the students scooted out except Jamie, who approached me while I packed up my notes. She said she had been reluctant to speak up in class because she would seem to be criticizing too many people she knows.

"I'm so glad you're looking into hooking up," she said. "I've always had a good head on my shoulders. I wasn't going to do anything stupid in college. But I certainly got caught up my first year in everything that was going on."

She told me she was a senior and currently in love with a boyfriend of more than two years. His name was Austin and he lived in her home city. My eyes lit up. Here was someone who could look back on her hooking-up experiences with the maturity that comes with age—and from the perspective of someone who had moved into something more permanent. We arranged to meet midafternoon the next day in the common room of a nearby dorm.

I got there early. Shafts of sunlight streamed through arched windows, giving the room the feel of a medieval cloister. Large, comfortable-looking couches and chairs, upholstered in neutral beiges and browns, showed no sign of recent use. Not another soul was present. There was a time when girls might have entertained guys in such a room, but that never happened anymore, Jamie would tell me later. Why should it, when students were free to lounge in the privacy of each other's rooms 'round the clock?

Jamie arrived precisely on time, striding across the room to shake my hand, a tall blonde dressed in a black Lacoste shirt and green linen skirt with tiny ruffles around the hem. Her hair was in a loose ponytail; her feet, toenails painted pink, were tucked into the rainbow flip-flops I had seen on other girls around campus. Everything about her, from those toenails to her gracefully erect posture, spoke of good breeding and self-control. I could see her living someday on Manhattan's Upper East Side and spending weekends in the Hamptons.

Parents of Duke's 6,500 undergraduates pay a lot of money annually to send their kids there—about $40,000 the year I observed Jamie. Although almost half of the students receive financial assistance, many students come from families of means, and Jamie, I would learn, was no exception. Her father worked in business overseas and earned enough money so that her mother, Ann, could be a full-time homemaker. Jamie and her brother grew up in a midsized city on the East Coast, doted on by Ann, who served them dinner every night and attended all their sporting competitions. Ann was an expert shopper, according to Jamie, and would spend days or weeks searching for exactly the right clothes, furnishings or other items Jamie might want at any given time. The weekend before I met Jamie, she had been missing Austin so much that her mother drove to Duke to take her to dinner and a movie. Some girls might have felt suffocated by so much attention, but Jamie didn't. She considered her mom a close friend and phoned her at least once a day, filling her in on her studies and friends.

"I'm lucky," she told me during that first interview. "I have so many friends who don't say 'I love you' to their parents."

Two things bothered her about her mother's life, however. As much as she benefited from Ann's attention, she didn't understand why her mother had stopped working outside the home once she had children. Ann had made her children her job; Jamie had no such plans. She wanted a career, she said, in media or film. She also wanted more romance in a marriage than what she saw at home; sparks should fly every time she and her husband saw each other, for years after they married.

High school had produced no golden boy but Duke did. Or so she thought when on a visit to the campus during her senior year in high school, she met a junior named Jake. Like her, he was tall and blond, "the hottest thing I'd ever seen." They had e-mailed each other over the summer before she arrived as a freshman in the fall. He contacted her once school began, and she started riding the campus bus from East to West several nights a week to visit him at his fraternity house. Social life at Duke revolved around the Greek system, and since fraternities had residential houses and sororities didn't, much of the action took place on the guys' territory.

Talking came easy to Jamie and Jake. They discussed sports, religion, even their philosophies of life with ease. He mentioned sharing a future with her and what they might name their kids. Although she knew not to take him seriously, the romantic in her loved these conversations.

Their leisure time, on the other hand, sounded dull at best. They spent most of it watching television at his fraternity and playing video games with his fraternity brothers. In late evening, they'd retire to bed and have sex. They never went to a movie and only once did Jake take her to dinner. Occasionally, they'd arrange to meet at a club and dance together, with the understanding that he could dance with other girls as well. He never offered to pick her up or take her home, even though his car was parked behind the frat house. She wrote it off as normal: "No other girls were getting rides."

Here was a girl who had been valued, by some standards indulged, all her life, crazy about a guy who played with her like a toy that had caught his eye. Looking back on that time, she could see that she was being used, but at the time she felt pretty good about herself. Duke students get to Duke by competing successfully against their peers, and that competitive spirit doesn't vanish as soon as they step on campus. In the minds of other freshman girls, Jake was quite a catch, which meant she was a winner.

Truth be told, she also didn't see any better options. Her connection to Jake, as one-sided as it appeared, was superior to the two alternatives she saw around campus. Her friend Lauren had chosen one of those options: a full-time boyfriend with whom she ate meals, took classes and spent the night. Such monogamous relationships—common on the Duke campus thirty years earlier—were scoffed at by other girls who had no desire to be what they called "joined at the hip" or "married" to anyone at this point in their lives. Another friend, Alison, had chosen a second path, hooking up randomly and frequently. She told Jamie "it was no big deal," because her partners always used condoms. Jamie wasn't drawn to that kind of action, either.

A month after school started, Jake backed away from Jamie, saying he wanted to "spend more time with his fraternity brothers." She found out he had been hooking up with other girls. While she had thought they were in love, he had merely considered her one of several hookup partners. She took this hard. Jake was the first man in college she had slept with, and even though the sex gave her no particular pleasure, she felt connected to him. Like many smart girls who believe they can have sex and not become emotionally attached, she was surprised by the depth of her feeling. Against her better judgment, she continued to seek him out that semester.

By her second semester, however, she was getting over him. She began playing the field, frequently at clubs such as Shooters, George's and Charlie's. These joints, a short drive from campus and independent of college control, were, by day, casual places for sandwiches and conversation. By eleven p.m., however, they morphed into bars with music so loud your ears rang for an hour once you left them. Jamie would flash her fake ID, have a couple of drinks and dance, either with her girlfriends or, as the night passed, with a guy. Occasionally, they would kiss while dancing, which the guy took as a signal that she was willing to go back to his room. It seemed awkward to turn him down, she recalled, given the fact that her friends had usually paired off already. Rather than be stranded, she'd go with the guy to his room and fool around in her underwear because it was easier to hook up than come up with a reason not to. She no longer recalls the names of most of these boys or even what they looked like. But she does remember being upset if, at the end of the night, they didn't ask for her phone number. She also remembers something else:

"The girls made all the effort. *The guys* didn't have to do anything."

In high school, Jamie had maintained more than a 4-point grade point average by taking Advanced Placement classes and been named an academic all-American. In her freshman year at Duke, her grades slid to a 2.5. By the time I met her, she had improved her academic performance considerably but was still puzzled by her earlier hookup behavior.

"If someone had told me in high school that I'd be doing that sort of stuff in a couple of years, I'd have said they were crazy," she admitted. She took comfort knowing she was far from the only one.

THE UN-RELATIONSHIP

Unless you've lived in a cave for the last couple of years, you've heard about hooking up, the most common way young people, male and female, straight and gay, relate intimately to each other, beginning as early as ages twelve and thirteen, and continuing into early adulthood. But what is it exactly?

It isn't exactly anything.

Hooking up can consist entirely of one kiss, or it can involve fondling, oral sex, anal sex, intercourse or any combination of those things. It can happen only once with a partner, several times during a week or over many months. Partners may know each other well, only slightly or not at all, even after they have hooked up regularly. A hookup often happens in a bedroom, although other places will do: dance floors, bars, bathrooms, auditoriums or any deserted room on campus. It is frequently unplanned, though it need not be. It can mean the start of something, the end of something or the whole something.

Feelings are discouraged, and both partners share an understanding that either of them can walk away at any time. Their behavior bewilders older generations, for they appear unhooked not only from guys but from our social expectations. Even those of us who didn't expect to find a marriage partner in college went there believing that our undergraduate years would deliver not only a great education but our first major, serious relationship, free of parental oversight. We looked forward to that. Young people today don't seem to feel that way. They talk about relationships, sure, but for the most part relationships that they can't afford or that didn't work out.

So how is hooking up different from what we used to call "casual sex"? Casual sex always meant intercourse—and it was the exception in college even during the '60s, '70s and early '80s, when most of these kids' parents were dating. Social historians now say that the "free love" phrase tossed around in the early part of that period characterized only a small proportion of young Americans. More girls didn't engage in casual sex than did, and if they did, they had to sneak around to do it lest they become known as promiscuous. With some exceptions, intercourse took place within a relationship that, at least on the young woman's part, implied some degree of commitment, and it followed several earlier stages of affection.

I was reminded of just how different things are today when, early in my research for this book, I was having dinner in San Francisco with a friend and her twenty-one-year-old stepdaughter, who had just graduated from a small state school. My friend was saying that in high school in the early 1970s, she "slept with" her boyfriend, "but only after going through the whole spectrum of behaviors, each of which signaled a new level of intimacy. We started with holding hands."

Her stepdaughter choked on the sip of water she had just taken. "You held hands?" she managed to say between coughs. "Oh my God, are you kidding me?"

None of this is meant to say that girls don't want to love and be loved, as Jamie did. But for reasons ranging from career plans to distrust of men, their prevailing philosophy is that love should wait, the result being that when, by what seems like accident or error, attachment occurs, they are torn up inside. Hooking up leaves them wholly unprepared for both the steadfastness and the flexibility a loving relationship requires.

To illustrate what hooking up can look like, let's return briefly to the dating that preceded it. A friend of mine, a Duke alumna in her early fifties, described a possible scene in a women's dorm at Duke early on a Tuesday evening in the fall of 1970:

The telephone rings at the switchboard, and a student operator, probably on a work-study grant, puts one finger on the page of the textbook she has been reading and with her other hand picks up the phone.

She listens for a couple of seconds and then switches on the microphone in front of her. "Susie Jenkins, telephone! Susie Jenkins, telephone!" Her no-nonsense voice sails through the dorm's public-address system, letting everyone in the dorm know that Susie may have a suitor.

Susie sprints down the hall to the phone at the end of the corridor. While other girls pop out of their rooms to make faces at her, she listens carefully and begins to smile. Frank, the frat boy in her European studies class, is calling to see if she'll go out with him on Saturday night. He asks if he can pick her up at her dorm at seven o'clock for dinner at The Ivy Room and later take her to the Sigma Chi party. She hesitates just long enough to let him squirm, and then accepts his invitation.

That Saturday, shortly before seven, she's in her room listening to the Carpenters sing "Close to You" on the radio when she hears the same receptionist's voice announcing, "Susie Jenkins, caller! Susie Jenkins, caller!" Susie asks her roommate to look over her outfit—a pink-and-gray plaid skirt and soft pink angora sweater—before heading out to meet Frank in the lobby. She signs his name in the registry at the desk and reminds him of the eleven p.m. curfew.

As excited as Susie is, she's also slightly nervous. She has never gone out with Frank before and has no idea how the two of them will get along. She sends up a silent prayer of thanks for the curfew system, grateful for the built-in excuse it provides if she isn't having a good time or Frank is having too good a time.

If she and Frank hit it off, they will know exactly what to expect as they progress from one date to the next, perhaps getting a little more sexual each time, maybe going steady. They may find a way eventually to sleep together when Susie's roommate is gone for the weekend, but such opportunities will be rare. Even in the next decade, as curfews were lifted and dorms went coed, the majority of Susies and Franks would have agreed that the goal of serious dating—and sex—was finding someone you wanted to be with permanently, or at least learning what it took to play for keeps.

Now fast-forward to fall of 2004 and a country-style saloon called Shooters a couple of miles from Duke in a gritty part of downtown Durham. The last stop before bed on a student's drunken weekend binge, it features dancing cages, a mechanical bull and dark, recessed corners. On this night, the disk jockey is spinning the hip-hop song "Back That Azz Up," and on the scuffed wooden dance floor, girls and guys are following the order, grinding their front- and backsides with one or two partners, known or unknown.

A sophomore we'll call Lindsay arrives with a bunch of girlfriends, flashes a fake ID to the bouncer outside and within a few minutes is sipping Smirnoff and tonic. She loves to dance and, once her drink is finished, is on the dance floor in her tight jeans and off-the-shoulder knit top, moving her torso and long, tanned arms seductively with the beat. Sometimes she dances with a female partner, sometimes alone.

Somewhere around one a.m., she spots a guy in khakis and a popped-collar Oxford shirt, which he wears, of course, with the sleeves pushed up to reveal his tan, muscular forearms. She knows his name is Adam, and not much else, but she likes what she sees and makes eye contact with him. He joins her on the dance floor for a short while and gradually they work their way over to a dark corner where they kiss and grope. He suggests that they get in her car and drive to her dorm, and she readily agrees. When they arrive at her room, she asks her roommate, Tasha, to find someplace else to sleep—a practice called "sexiling"—and Tasha agrees because at some point, she'll want to ask the same thing of Lindsay.

Lindsay and Adam have sex. Adam, like many guys, keeps a couple of condoms in his wallet for times like this. Eventually, he leaves. She has no idea whether she'll go out with him again or whether she even wants to.

That afternoon, a girlfriend asks her what she did the previous night: "Did you hook up or *hook up*?"

That's the beauty of the term "hooking up" for girls: It's so vague that they can do whatever they want and not feel bad or even awkward when dishing with a girlfriend. Despite wanting to appear cool, they may still feel like used goods after a night in the sack. As one college professor explained, "Saying 'I hooked up last night with this guy whose name I don't remember' is a lot easier than saying 'I gave this guy whose name I don't remember a blow job last night.'"

You've got to give them credit; they've come up with a vocabulary that gives them maximum freedom. The distance between what one says and what one means has never been greater. They don't have boyfriends and girlfriends; they have "friends with benefits" or, to confuse classmates even more, just "friends." They don't go on dates but may say they're dating someone. They also may be "talking to" someone but not "having a conversation" unless it's serious. If they declare themselves a couple and then argue over something, they may "go on a break" and hook up with other partners while they decide whether to resume the relationship. If they leave high school for different colleges, they may declare themselves neither finished nor faithful but in an "open relationship," meaning both of them can be "sort of seeing" someone else on the side.

When they actually describe intimate encounters, they do so in terms of performance—and how well they perform—rather than how they feel about what they're doing or why they chose to do it. A girl will say she "teabagged" a guy, meaning she took his testicles into her mouth. A guy will say he "had a roast beef sandwich" if he went down on a girl.

Like past generations, these young people enjoy making up words to describe the aspects of their sexual culture that only they are meant to understand, such as "shack pack" (toothbrushes, toothpaste and other supplies given to pledges by sororities), "horority" (sorority), and the "roll and scream" when, according to one female Dukie, "you roll over the next morning so horrified at what you find next to you that you scream."

It's hard not to laugh at their colorful language, and equally hard not to be a bit disturbed by the attitude that intimacy is disposable. Teachers remark on this frequently. "There's always been a lot of sex in college," says Harvard University psychologist Mark O'Connell. "It's the quality of sex that's changed. It's increasingly disconnected."

Robin Sawyer, a public-health professor who teaches a popular human sexuality course at the University of Maryland, surveyed three hundred students, asking what hooking up means. "My favorite response," he recalls, "was 'random oral sex.' I said, 'What the hell does that mean? You walk into the student union and say I'll pick every third boy or girl I see?' I've been teaching for over twenty years and seen a lot of pushing the envelope. This hanging out and hooking up has been a trip for me."

"Come on," some students say to such comments. "We use condoms." (And indeed they do, more frequently than past generations.) "Can't we just enjoy sex without grown-ups getting on our case? Sex without love may be meaningless, but on the list of meaningless things that are fun, it's pretty high up there." Two students in the sexuality class I taught at George Washington University, a guy and a girl, made this point one evening. Tony, a junior from New York, had earlier described himself as a "man-whore." Sacha was also a junior.

Eleven of us were sitting around a conference table in a small library. Tony began:

"There's a girl who calls me when we're both single, just because she likes to have sex with me. Nothing else. I could never have a conversation with her if I wanted to. It was just purely . . . the time is right to be havin' some sex. And . . . the next day I'll see her on the street and it's, 'Hey, what's goin' on?' And that's it."

He continued, "I was the one who actually stopped the whole situation. Because I was baffled. It was mind-boggling. I'd try to talk to her, I'd be like, 'Hey . . . wanna talk about something?' She never did."

Sacha picked up the discussion.

"I hooked up with a guy on and off for a year, and I don't think we ever had a conversation. Like, really, it was just, like, 'See you later.' And it was fun. I mean we both had a good time."

Several "Yeahs" and "Mm-hmms" were heard around the table.

Hooking up first surfaced as a sexual concept in porn magazines in the early 1990s. Within a few years, the term had made its way onto college campuses across the United States, starting with the pricey private schools. "Everyone here seems intent on hooking up as fast as possible," a freshman at Columbia University told National Public Radio in 1996. A year later, in 1997, a Brown University student told *The New York Times*, "In a normal relationship, you meet, get drunk, hook up." A major research project on gender issues at Duke, led by undergraduates and supervised by faculty during the 2002–2003 school year, reported that "students rarely go on formal dates but instead attend parties in large groups, followed by 'hook-ups'—unplanned sexual encounters fueled by alcohol."

Social trends such as hooking up may start with privileged kids, but they're rarely confined to one class. In 2000, Elizabeth Paul, a professor at the College of New Jersey (formerly a teacher's college known as Trenton State), surveyed 555 undergrads and found that almost four out of five students had hooked up; half said they started their evenings planning to have some form of sex, with no particular person in mind. A study a couple of years later at James Madison University in Virginia, with 15,000 students, reported similar proportions, one at the University of Wisconsin, whose undergraduates number about 28,000, only slightly less. In my own reporting in the Washington, D.C.–Baltimore corridor, I've talked about hooking up with students on campuses as diverse as the

University of the District of Columbia, a predominantly black com-
muter school, and Towson University, a residential state college just
north of Baltimore.

Certainly, traditional dating can be found on campuses as well, particularly those with active religious affiliations or located in the South.
As Jessica, a student from Atlanta in my GW class, told me, "My girlfriends at Auburn, Savannah College of Art and Design and Georgia
Southern seem to always go on dates and then date boys for longer periods of time." But at many other colleges and universities, dating is like
an elderly aunt who sits alone and forgotten at the dining table rather than
a lively guest next to whom everyone wants to sit.

Accounts in the late 1990s of hooking up in college were followed by
reports, first in *The Washington Post* and later in other national publica-
tions, that it had surfaced in high schools and even some middle schools,
with girls as young as twelve and thirteen saying they had given blow jobs
to boys. This shouldn't have surprised anyone: Sexual trends among
older youths, once established, tend to be imitated by younger kids. At
the time, little data existed to expand on these accounts because squeam-
ish federal bureaucrats, who dole out most of the dollars for research on
sexuality, had told surveyors *not* to ask about oral sex, anal sex, heavy petting or sex with a homosexual partner—in short, most of the sexual behaviors included in the catch-all phrase "hooking up."

Scientists in the 1990s did, however, start noticing a first-ever decline
in dating among high school students of all racial, ethnic and income
groups. Researchers at Bowling Green State University in Ohio picked
up something else as well among Toledo-area students: Of the fifty-five
percent of eleventh-graders who reported having intercourse, one-third
said it was with someone who was only a friend, not a boyfriend or girlfriend. Presumably, the proportion would have been higher if the survey
had included sexual activities other than intercourse.

In mid-2005, a study funded by the Centers for Disease Control and

Prevention (CDC) gave credence to these unofficial reports of early sexual behavior. Figures showed that while the percentage of high school students having intercourse was declining slightly, those who did have sex were starting at a younger age. This was particularly true for girls— and tipped me off to the fact that in public conversations, we were missing a significant point: Hooking up—or more precisely, unhooking— might have been just a footnote in social history, the curious behavior of a promiscuous few, had it not fit so neatly into the new lives young women were creating.

SHIFTING THE BALANCE OF POWER

In the courtship tradition of late-nineteenth- and early-twentieth-century America, women ran the show. Mothers would first invite young men to call on their daughters on specified days and at specified times. In the following months, according to social historian Beth Bailey, a young woman could issue her own invitations to young men to whom she had been formally introduced elsewhere. Visits still took place in the home, usually with her mother presiding. It was considered improper, in those days, for a young man to ask to call on a young woman. Young women were, back then, proactors.

The subsequent convention of dating changed them to reactors. Dating, says Bailey, came about in the early 1900s as a response of the lower social classes to crowded living conditions. "Calling" simply wasn't practical when you shared a one- or two-room flat with four or more people. Working-class women didn't usually have parlors, so they began to seek out the streets, dance halls and eventually the movies as places to meet their beaus. Middle- and upper-class young women, attracted by the idea of being out from under a mother's eye, soon sought the same freedom. But given the parental restraints of the times, they couldn't appear too eager or, heaven forbid, ask to leave the house on their own. Thus evolved the tradition of boys asking girls to go "out." Boys were expected to pick up girls at home, take them out and pay all expenses. By 1925, dating had become common, and it became increasingly so over the next few decades as more and more families purchased automobiles.

In her book *From Front Porch to Back Seat,* Bailey contends that by taking control of the date, and moving the place of courtship from the woman's sphere of the home to the man's sphere of the outside world, men were buying not only female companionship but power. "Men asked women out; women were condemned as 'aggressive' if they expressed interest in a man too directly," Bailey writes. "Men paid for everything, but often with the implication that women 'owed' sexual favors in return. The dating system required men always to assume control, and women to act as men's dependents." This held true until the late 1960s, when the women's movement began to forcefully challenge dating's assumptions.

Within both courtship and dating, girls' one real area of control was sex. They could set and enforce limits on how far a boy could go. They became known as the sexual gatekeepers, but their power wasn't absolute. A "No" could be overridden, sometimes brutally so, and as gatekeepers, they took much if not all of the blame when that happened.

Of course, from a man's perspective, a woman back then possessed a great deal of power. If girls resented being at the mercy of boys to make the first move, boys worried that their first moves would be rejected, sometimes harshly. Girls and boys worked out conventions to disguise her assertiveness and reduce the likelihood of his being rejected. Flirtation, casual banter and, especially, mutual friends as messengers were used to start the mating dance and move it along.

For about ten years, beginning in the early 1920s, a group of young women very much like the current generation tried to reclaim the power they believed women had lost. The flappers—so called because of the fashion of wearing unbuckled galoshes that flapped as the women walked—were energetic and daring. Daughters of a well-to-do, educated middle class, they shocked people by flying airplanes and driving cars, chopping off their hair and hiking up their skirts, inviting young men on dates rather than waiting for young men to call, drinking in public and holding petting parties. While their mothers had devoted themselves to securing voting rights, organizing unions and establishing urban settlement houses, the flappers, writes author Gail Collins, "were interested in a different form of liberation—the kind that gave them the right to enjoy themselves in the same ways men did. . . . The new national pastimes were necking and petting—terms that seemed to cover behavior ranging from nuzzling to everything short of intercourse. . . . The underlying impulse was freedom—from the mores of the past that required women to keep themselves in check, physically and emotionally."

That freedom disappeared as the old norms reasserted themselves under the weight of the Depression, economic hardship and a conservative cultural backlash. But by the 1960s, freedom returned in the form of women's liberation, which demanded, as the flappers had, equality on the job and in the bedroom. Today's young women, urged to be bold from the time they could talk and walk, have assumed the same mandate. Depending on your point of view, they're either mimicking male behavior—a kind of "I'll see your bet and raise you one"—or enjoying their bodies in ways their mothers never did. Freedom to be openly sexual has leveled the playing field for some girls; they don't have to be pretty and popular to attract guys, nor do they have to worry as much as past generations did about acquiring a (bad) reputation.

Statistics confound the once common assumption that boys are hunters and girls are prey. In one study, young women fifteen to twenty-four were *less* likely than young men to say they felt pressured to engage in intercourse. Recent federal research also shows that the proportion of girls having sex before age fifteen is the same proportion as boys; that more girls than boys now have intercourse from the time they turn sixteen until they graduate from high school; and that the proportion of high school girls who report having one-night stands, as well as nonromantic sexual relationships, equals that of boys. These percentages account for less than half the survey group, but that quickly changes in college.

The popular impression that young women couldn't possibly pursue sex for their own pleasure still hangs on, however. A great example was the media hoo-ha over the 2005 CDC report, possibly the agency's most comprehensive survey ever on sexual behavior, showing a high incidence of oral sex among all ages surveyed. Columnists opined at length about how terrible it was that so many young women were servicing young men. In their view, the double standard was still alive and well.

What writers missed was that in the same survey, young women reported *receiving* oral sex in virtually the same numbers as young men. There was nothing to indicate their overall satisfaction, however.

Of course, hooking up gives guys something as well, and it's a big something: more immediate access to sex without having to work for it. One can argue that that helps explain its popularity. As Jamie's experience with Jake illustrated so poignantly—and as other girls in my book confirmed—guys frequently create the social environment in which hooking up flourishes and set the expectations about what girls will do. Some older feminists have even suggested that men use the hookup as revenge against women they believe are moving ahead of them in school and careers.

Whether spurred on by nefarious motives or simply enjoying the freedom of uncensored lust, guys have no doubt that they're the winners in the hookup culture. "Because girls are more assertive, it's easy for us to be assholes," a senior man at GW told me.

What puzzles older adults, and even girls themselves when they're being honest, is why incredibly smart, talented and seemingly confident young women would let themselves be used when what they're doing isn't making them particularly happy.

Females' sexual assertiveness mirrors—and, I would argue, stems partly from—what they've shown in classrooms and on the playing field. In 1980, about the time many of them were born, the proportion of females enrolled in college exceeded the proportion of males for the first time in American history, 52 to 48 percent. By 1990, when these young women were approaching or in elementary school, the gap had widened—55 to 45 percent. In that same year, female enrollment in graduate schools jumped over that of males.

Girls continued to outnumber—and outpace—their brothers and male friends all the way through school. By 1998, virtually the same percentages of them were taking math and science courses in high school, and more of them were taking Advanced Placement exams. By the 2001–2002 academic year, women were earning more associate's, bachelor's and master's degrees than men. In that same year, Harvard Medical School enrolled its first majority-female class; the next fall, Yale Law School followed suit. In May 2005, Creighton University School of Medicine, a Jesuit school in Omaha, graduated fifty-four women and fifty-one men. Even the Duke report on gender, critical of male dominance in several areas of campus life, including student government, concluded that equality prevailed in the classroom.

Girls have accomplished similar success in sports. While discrepancies in resources still exist, the change in the number and quality of female athletes—in a little over one generation—is astounding. When Congress, in 1972, passed Title IX, the law prohibiting discrimination in schools based on gender, about 300,000 girls played high school sports, or one in twenty-seven. Now that figure approaches 3 million, or about one in three. Girls take part in virtually all sports that boys do, challenging the guys in the number of state and national championships they bring back to their high schools and colleges. Thousands of individual girls play on male teams. A few have gone on to compete against men in professional golf, hockey and even Division I-A football.

More than half of the girls in this book played at least one sport, and all of those who did excelled. Sienna, for example, played on the field hockey team of her Washington-area high school, a team known as one of the best in the area. Cleo's basketball team competed in the Texas state championship when she was a senior. Alicia's bedroom in high school was decorated with more than seventy medals from district, regional and state gymnastics tournaments.

Since hooking up is relatively new and its characteristics are not easily captured in survey questions, there has been little research on the possible reasons for girls' sexual assertiveness. One line of thinking says that when females outnumber males on, say, a college campus, they have to compete with whatever resources they possess, including their bodies. Another idea, intriguing but not proven conclusively, proposes that women who pursue challenging mental tasks develop higher levels of testosterone, the hormone linked to a strong competitive drive in all facets of life, including sex.

The behavior and words of the girls I've observed suggest another, two-part theory: From the time they could walk, they've been told by parents and other adults, in subtle and not-so-subtle ways, not only that they *can* go for what they want, but that they *should*. They have taken this message to heart, been roundly acclaimed for their good grades and trophies—and carried the same attitude into the bedroom. As Sienna, the private high school sophomore, told me, "Who says girls can't play guys just like guys have always played girls?"

The second part of my theory is this: In order to accomplish the goals that their parents—and by this time in their lives, they—want, they believe they can't afford to invest time, energy and emotion in a deep relationship. Hooking up appears to be a practical alternative.

They have a point. The interval between when a girl enters puberty and when she marries keeps expanding to—as I write this—an average of more than thirteen years. That's a long time to wait to have sex. Hooking up enables a young woman to practice a piece of a relationship, the physical, while devoting most of her energy to staying on the honor roll, being accepted into a well-known university and then keeping up her academic scholarship while working ten or fifteen hours a week in the cafeteria, playing lacrosse, working out every day in the gym and applying to graduate programs in engineering. She's nothing if not obedient.

Of course, as Jamie learned, hooking up can damage one's psyche and grades. But it doesn't have to, and it's easy to think you can handle it, particularly if, with the help of adoring parents, you've been able to manage everything else in your life until that point. They're on a roll, these young women, determined to do as well or better in college than they did in high school and to land great jobs. More than their mothers, they believe that once they get out of college and are on their own—a longer transition than it used to be, lasting into the mid- to late twenties— they will be supporting themselves financially, possibly without substantial assistance from a husband. They can't blow college.

Julie, a GW senior, put it this way: "I don't have time or energy to worry about a 'we.' "

Young women tell researchers the same thing the Duke class told me: that they do eventually want to be married and have children. But they also voice significant concerns about whether they can do both well and enjoy a successful career. Some say that being single may be just as satisfying. Others fantasize about choosing their wedding dresses and bridesmaids but don't plan to find the groom until their late twenties or early thirties. Some in that latter group see no reason to practice being a loving partner before then. Or, if they have a partner, they refuse to call him their boyfriend.

"You have plenty of time to fall in love later," parents tell them, and they believe it. Hooking up wouldn't have become mainstream if it didn't appeal to them as useful, even necessary, in achieving what they want and what others want for them. They hope to make their mark, so they mark their time with relationships that are going nowhere, making up the rules and vocabulary as they go along.

In essence, they have analyzed the benefits and costs of relationships and come up with what they think is a bargain.

If they were to date someone seriously, they'd enjoy steady companionship, affection and perhaps an occasional bauble or bouquet. But the costs would be enormous: time that could be spent with friends, attention to schoolwork or athletics and, perhaps the most significant, a cost to their sense of independence. They're also not stupid, these girls. They've watched their parents' marriage, or marriages, and what they see can appear fractious or, at best, as in Jamie's case, dull. If that's what a long-term relationship looks like, who in her right, bright mind would want that, at least while you're young?

Scholars now know some general things about how marriage affects children. Children growing up in a two-parent home where there is minimal conflict tend to have fewer problems in school and with friends than those who live with one parent. They also tend to wait longer to have sex for the first time and are more likely to say they want to be married someday.

But does postponing first-time intercourse by a year or so mean a girl hooks up less frequently? I doubt it. Is the girl who says she wants to be married more likely to seek monogamous, long-term relationships in her youth? Not necessarily.

One subject girls talked about a lot was the power their mothers either had or didn't have with the girls' fathers, or, in one girl's case, a stepfather. Their mothers tended to either depend a lot on their husbands, financially and emotionally, or be completely independent. Marriage as a true partnership, particularly an affectionate partnership, seemed an elusive concept. From what they saw at home, to tell a man "I need you" was like saying "I'm incomplete without you." A young man might say that and sound affectionate, they said. But to an ambitious young woman, who had been taught from childhood to define power on her terms and defend it against all comers, need signaled weakness.

An instant-message conversation that took place between Shaida, a Duke sophomore, and a girlfriend who thought she was falling in love brought this home to me:

GIRLFRIEND: and we layed [sic] in bed and talked for like four hours and like had sex during the whole thing; it was really like a moment; like he held me sooo tight for the rest of the night; i woke up like really close to him; and i felt something. . . .

SHAIDA: that's incredible intimacy . . . do you love him?

GIRLFRIEND: i am scared of loving him

SHAIDA: because of what being in love will do to you

GIRLFRIEND: because of what does that say about me. . . . i'm just a weepy girl who relies on someone. . . . i want to be independent and i think that it is important for women of our generation but by saying i love someone and need him it's like contradictory . . . hypocritical . . . but i also don't want to give into love because i am scared he won't call me. . . . and i will be heartbroken and then feel like a stupid girl that should have known better.

Even for girls who do enter into relationships, it is not a coincidence that they not only eschew such labels as "boyfriend" and "girlfriend" but also the tokens that, in their parents' generation, used to accompany these words. To them, rings and fraternity pins signal not so much deep affection and abiding interest as a young man's claim on his territory.

The truth is that some of these girls see themselves as winners in almost everything else in their lives and fear they might be losers when it comes to love. Cleo, a senior at GW, was starting to go out with Steven when she put it quite colorfully: "It will suck if it's bad, but it will suck even more if it's good." Leah, a gay junior coming out of a couple of short-term relationships, complained, "Serial monogamy is exhausting. You put all your emotions into a relationship, and then you have to do it all over again." She was ready to start hooking up again because it allowed her to check her feelings at the bedroom door, or at least pretend to, saving her psychic energy for the other dramas of her busy life.

Alicia, a junior at Duke, felt the same way at one point. "Sex is more tangible than love," she wrote. "And it is much, much easier than taking the time to know someone. Real relationships must be integrated into a much more complex set of goals and life objectives. It's safer to get your sex and acceptance through something short-term and unserious."

THE ENABLERS

The deal that young women have struck wouldn't last without the support of backers, some of them unwitting. As journalist and social critic Malcolm Gladwell points out in his book *The Tipping Point*, small changes in a population become trends, or "tip," as a result of cultural prompts, many of them small or subtle.

One of those prompts is supplied by girls themselves. Traditionally, women, young and old, have been the main voices telling other women to play hard to get and slow down. Girls today largely accept hooking up, if not for themselves personally, for other girls. Some girls, such as Jamie, say they hook up primarily because their girlfriends do.

Girls hear their mothers' voices as well but the messages they *hear*, as opposed to the messages their mothers probably intend to convey, sometimes discourage them from seeking serious relationships. Julie, the GW senior who didn't have time for a "we," told me about her mother finding her in the kitchen when she was fifteen, sobbing over a boyfriend of two years.

"What's wrong?" Mom asked.

"Bill just broke up with me," Julie said.

Mom rolled her eyes and walked out of the room. "At your age," she said over her shoulder, "you don't need a boyfriend." Julie remembered that encounter six years earlier as if it had just happened. What she took away from it was that her mother didn't think relationships at her age, or love for that matter, were very important.

A high school senior I interviewed remembered her mother telling her, "You don't have to be with a guy to be valued." The mom was right, of course, but she failed her daughter by not telling her also that she could be with a guy and still feel valued, though it wasn't having a boyfriend that made her valuable. As far as sowing a seed about the wisdom of youthful committed relationships, these moms' castoff remarks, and others that followed, trumped everything else their daughters heard, saw or read. In survey after survey, teens say parents influence their decisions about relationships and sex more than anyone else, including their friends.

Parents who play down their kids' early crushes may be worried that the crushes will lead to sex and possibly disease or pregnancy. These are legitimate concerns that need parental attention. But girls should not be denied the opportunity to have these crushes and talk about them. Early relationships, even when they go sour, teach girls important things about love. Better that a girl work through such first-time emotions with her parents' support than on her own later.

Ideally, girls would enjoy that support from both mother and father. In reality, when they get it, it almost always comes from the mother or another older woman. Although American fathers appear to be spending more time with their daughters than they used to, that is true primarily in their daughters' early years. Fathers and adolescent daughters do less together than fathers and sons, mothers and daughters, and mothers and sons. Would they do more if they knew that their daughters might drink less often, start dating later and begin sex later if they paid more attention? That's what the research shows. I frankly don't know if it would change their behavior. What I do know for all the girls in this book, as well as those in my last book, is that Mom's was the primary voice. And that when pressed, girls admitted wishing for more time with, and attention from, their dads. I'll never forget watching one girl prepare to leave her house for a formal dance at school. Her date and his parents had arrived, camera in hand. Her mom was passing around soft drinks. Her dad arrived from his son's soccer match and passed through the room without giving a glance at his gorgeous daughter. When I mentioned this to her later, she shrugged. Normally a chatterbox, she didn't say a word.

Both mothers and fathers of the girls in this book wanted the best for their daughters: the best schools, the best grades, the best jobs. The best partners? I would ask them. Of course, they'd reply, but first things first. Cleo and her sister Nicole, both students at GW, had gotten that message loud and clear from both parents. At an early dinner on campus, one of the first things they told me about was the newspaper quote their mother taped to their desks at home when they were in elementary school: "How much you earn is determined by how much you learn." When I visited their home months later, I saw that the quote was still up in their rooms.

Parents aren't the only adults who sometimes act as if they fear girls are going to elope with the first good-looking man they meet. Shaida told of her high school commencement speaker's final words; she had pasted it on the last page of her high school scrapbook in order not to forget it. "A message to all you girls," the man had said. "Get educated. Find a career. Be self-sufficient. And then find Prince Charming." Shaida and her classmates apparently had a choice: They could either achieve or love. They shouldn't try to do both at once.

As important as what kids hear from adults is what they don't hear. For example, evidence suggests that comprehensive sex education in middle and high school delays sexual activity and reduces teen pregnancies and sexually transmitted diseases. But as Jamie pointed out to me, instructors sometimes assume sex happens only with a boyfriend, or they feel comfortable talking about sex only within a committed relationship. "They say things like 'Make your decisions together,' " she recalled. "That's not the real world. Hookups can occur on the spur of the moment, without much conversation. [Teachers] need to stress that the unexpected can happen to smart people."

And if teachers don't say enough about casual sex in secondary school, college faculty and administrators are virtually mute; witness the GW date auction described earlier in which students stripped to their barest essentials while college personnel looked on. Campus women's centers sponsor sexuality workshops that provide students with useful information about health issues as well as pleasure, but spend little time discussing the merits of, and problems with, relationships. Once girls step on a college campus, they may quickly get the idea that everyone there is having sex and plenty of it—and that it's just fine with their elders.

Adolescents are the most social of human beings. They adopt the behavior and attitudes of the people closest to them. Their head is telling them that no-strings sex, whether intercourse or simply the warm-up exercises, makes sense. Their bodies and their friends are saying, "Go for it." Parents and other adults are steering them away from committed relationships.

Why wouldn't they hook up?

A SEA OF SEXUAL IMAGES

When Jamie was brooding over boys, she would watch "reality" TV shows about dating such as *The Bachelorette* and take heart at the show's crop of gorgeous men eager to squire women around. When Shaida, also at Duke, was bummed out over a hookup, she would play the defiant lyrics of feminist songstress Ani DiFranco on her computer as she got ready to go out and try again. Nicole, angered by a particularly annoying guy, would trash him on her computer by typing an in-your-face "away" message on her AOL account that any of the 240 people on her message list could read and respond to.

Although neither as benign as supporters say nor as harmful as the critics would have us believe, the media play an unprecedented role today in shaping girls' views on their romantic and sexual lives. Given the fact that older adults are reluctant to discuss issues of intimacy other than, perhaps, the mechanics of, and morality surrounding, sex, it shouldn't surprise us that young people turn to the media for education and guidance in the area of life they arguably think more about than any other.

Researchers estimate that before reaching college, American adolescents spend about eight hours a day listening to recorded music, watching TV, going to the movies, using the Internet and reading magazines. Sexuality and sex have been part of the media sea in which kids have been swimming since the 1970s, and the amount of sexual imagery has undeniably increased. A study of shows watched by adolescents, released in 2002, reported that four out of five programs contained sexual material. A 2005 study revealed that the number of sexual scenes on television had doubled since 1998. The 2005 study also reported that the percentage of scenes showing characters having sex after they had just met had doubled between 2002 and 2005.

With each year, it seems, the sexual sea swells. R-rated movies, according to one study, contain seven times as many sexual acts or references as television, and intercourse between two unmarried people is thirty-two times more likely to happen on film than on TV. Some, though not all, music videos on MTV rival explicit movies in the nature and amount of sexual content. The first pop heroines for women in college today were Britney Spears and Christina Aguilera.

We needn't get overly alarmed about this. Media do not cause young people to do certain things; most girls and guys, according to recent studies, do not simply ape what they see. Instead, young people react to, and use, media based on the kind of people they already are and hope to become. On TV, the movie screen and the Web, they see people their age and older who look or act in ways that they would like to adopt or avoid, and they take special interest in what Jane Brown, a professor of media studies at the University of North Carolina, calls sexual and romantic scripts. We can learn what kind of relationships they would like, in addition to what they have, by paying attention to their favorite shows and movies.

One of their favorites is *Laguna Beach*, MTV's racy series about a group of high school students in Orange County, California. In one highly rated episode, the show's female hotties hinted to favored guys that they expected to be invited to their prom in extraordinary ways. And so they were. Invitations from boys appeared at the end of scavenger hunts, tucked into dozens and dozens of roses or written across a chocolate cake presented at an expensive restaurant. This was pure, old-fashioned courting the series' girls were demanding—if a bit over the top—and the reaction of female fans was telling. All across America that year and the next, junior and senior girls in high school asked for, and received, the same treatment from real boys, indicating how, deep inside, many girls long to be wooed.

The Fox network's *The OC*, a nighttime soap opera about two high school couples and their families, also set in Orange County, is popular with college students as well as teens not just because it stars great-looking characters living in palatial houses by the sea but because Seth and Summer, Ryan and Marissa (until she was killed) appear to really care for each other. Adults may decry the sex in the show (actually, after the first season, there wasn't that much) and not recognize the tension, tenderness and, yes, deep love portrayed between the couples. It's also noteworthy that although hookups occur occasionally, this show is principally about relationships—including the demonstrably loving, if occasionally rocky, marriage of Sandy and Kirsten, the starring father and mother.

Magazines also help young women sort through affairs of the heart; almost three out of four teenaged girls say they read them regularly. Like other forms of media, they act like a good friend might, explaining the popular culture and suggesting ways to fit in. A half-hour spent scanning a newsstand tells a lot about how the commercial interests of New York and Los Angeles think young women should act around young men: part aggressor, part supplicant, rarely the partner. *Cosmopolitan,* the most popular magazine among college-aged women, is particularly prone to extremes. One issue, to give a random example, carried articles titled: "Boost His Body Confidence!" "A Dinner He'll Die For!" "When He Moves On Before You Do!" "Clue In to His Carnal Cravings!" Nothing in this issue suggested what a woman might expect a man to do for her.

As powerful as traditional media are, they do not possess nearly the authority that friends do—influence that has expanded exponentially with the growth of new media: computer e-mails, instant messages, chat rooms and cell phones. Ninety percent of adolescents in high-income families have a computer at home, and so do eighty percent in less-well-off families. More than half of older adolescents and young adults own mobile phones, a proportion that is growing rapidly, particularly among teenaged girls. Wired and wireless communication enable, and indeed encourage, young women and young men to talk to each other out of view of their parents, arranging encounters of various kinds and then analyzing them for days afterward. Long gone are the days when Mom or Dad could answer the phone and ask, "Who's calling, please?"

Work at the University of Southern California has shown that a significant majority of young people now make most of their social engagements through digital means. Text messages and instant messages are not only convenient and private but enable girls and guys to make bold suggestions at the last minute—and terminate further relationships without the emotion of face-to-face conversation.

It is not unusual for young women to type more than a thousand text messages a month on their cell phones. My husband and I observed such a girl in action one Saturday night when we were out for dinner at a pricey restaurant. A couple about our age, newly married and each with two daughters, was celebrating their special day at the table next to us. Three of the four daughters, who looked to be in their late teens, chatted away with the adults. The fourth daughter we had our eye on, also a teenager, chimed in occasionally but focused most of her attention on a cell phone in her lap, discreetly hidden in the folds of her skirt. As she monitored the face of her phone for text messages and tapped in her replies, I couldn't help but wonder whether she was arranging to meet someone.

LOVE, THE INSISTENT BYSTANDER

When a girl believes that she cannot risk her time, emotions or independence on commitment, hookups are an easy substitute in which the benefits outweigh the costs—until someone comes along who takes her breath away. Then she simultaneously wants to hold on tightly and run away as fast as she can. No matter how much she resists, she finds herself thinking only about the person she hopes will be her partner. Neuroscience is teaching us that her reactions, based in her biology, are not just the fantasy of poets but also nature's way, long ago, of making sure our species survived.

Romantic love insists on developing, even in the world of casual sex. Four of the six girls I observed at Duke and GW—and all of the high school girls—hooked up during the school year that I observed. Sex, in whatever form they chose, was easy to get and easy to give away. They tried not to become attached, but some ended up feeling attached anyway.

Several of them also had deeper relationships, which, though not long-lasting, both complicated and enriched their lives. They had been trying to avoid love for fear it would get in the way of their ambitions and plans and everyone's expectations, including their own. They had been running from the idea of a real relationship because they worried they might not be good at it or it wouldn't last and they would get hurt. They discovered that some of their fears were true. But they also learned that to be cherished and to cherish in return were feelings like no other.

Little in their lives had prepared them for what lay ahead once they found themselves in love. There were so many sensations coming at them at the same time: The pleasure of being admired. The comfort of having someone to turn to. The distress of separation. The worry that came with cheating or being cheated on. There were priorities they'd have to rearrange, choices they'd have to make. And, oh, the questions: Was this a passionate but short-lived infatuation, or long-lasting love? Could they be committed to someone for a while without promising a long-term future? How should they talk to a partner who might see the relationship differently than they did or want different things from it? They had only friends and the media to turn to for answers.

Their mothers might have had "the sex talk" with them but, with the exception of Jamie's and Sienna's mothers, had not talked much about love. And what they saw between their mothers and fathers was not particularly helpful. Several girls told me that they had heard their parents say they loved each other. But like Jamie, they had rarely seen Mom and Dad kiss, hug, act playfully or appear to enjoy each other's company. Three girls, two in high school, one in college, had witnessed dreadful fighting between parents who eventually divorced. Love, to them, seemed an awful lot like marriage: sometimes risky, frequently boring and potentially very hurtful.

Their confusion was understandable. Unlike other nationalities, Americans use the word "love" for so many things—new friends, comfy old bathrobes, the coffee shop down the street—that it has become virtually meaningless. For much of the last century, outside Hollywood movies, the concept of romantic love, along with tenderness, patience and thoughtfulness, has lost much of its luster. Even Dr. Phil rarely mentions it. For these young women to admit that they were in love, particularly in the highly charged professional world in which their parents worked and to which they aspired, was to open themselves up to accusations of softness and muddy-headedness.

The sidelining of love in our culture is fairly recent. Stories of love, both mythological and historical, are plentiful; one survey found evidence of passion in almost ninety percent of the 166 varied societies that were studied. In the nineteenth and early twentieth centuries, romance was embraced by American men as well as women, as evidenced in letters from Nathaniel Hawthorne to Sophia Peabody, poet Paul Laurence Dunbar to Alice Ruth Moore and Albert Einstein to Mileva Marić.

But by the 1930s, scientists were declaring love the stuff of childhood fantasies and sentimental women. Psychotherapist Alfred Adler was one such critic, denouncing romantic ideals as outdated, even unhealthy, and arguing in *Esquire* magazine for rational, cooperative marriages that aimed for companionship rather than emotional connectedness.

As I watched young women, in between hookups and periods of solitude, attempt something bordering on relationships, I thought about how we usually learn to love in stages, becoming a better lover (not just a better "sexer" or "screwer") as we get to know our partner. Good love demands paying attention to the other, talking honestly and, most of all, taking the time required to learn how to do those things. Dating in the mid-twentieth century was far from perfect training, but it did build relationships over weeks or months or sometimes even years. A great deal of learning took place or at least had the opportunity to take place. Parents talked even less about sex and love back then, but there were norms that gave girls at least some idea of what they could or should do. We might have rebelled against some of those conventions—I certainly did—but, like Susie Jenkins and her curfew in 1970, we also had something to fall back on when our little revolts blew up in our faces.

When I think of girls learning to love, I picture them floating in a large, turbulent sea, treading water but unable to get to shore because they have never learned how to swim. Without the conventions of dating, when today's girls fall in love, they don't know how to move the relationship forward. And when love doesn't materialize, or disappears, they become deeply depressed at losing their partner and the self-control they have spent most of their young lives constructing.

JAMIE, IN LOVE

Jamie met Austin, her first love, one night at a friend's house in her hometown the summer after her freshman year at Duke. He attended a state university several hundred miles away, was a year ahead of her in school and had dark-brown hair, deep-blue eyes, an inquiring mind and outgoing personality. He asked her out to a movie for the next evening.

"I was like, A date? What is going on?" she told me during our first conversation in the dorm. To her surprise, she got very nervous waiting for him to pick her up.

Austin, in a separate interview, described their first meeting in glowing terms. As a high school senior, he had had his heart broken by a girlfriend who cheated on him. He didn't take relationships seriously after that, and spent much of his free time in his freshman and sophomore years hooking up with "ten or twenty girls." He told me he was surprised how "easy" the girls at his school were, how they would "just give stuff away before they even knew the person." That first night with Jamie, he could tell right away that she was classier than the girls he'd been hanging out with and not likely to throw herself at him.

She was equally impressed with him. "We spent the whole night talking," she recalled. "He wanted to know what I liked to do, places I'd been.

It was a really cool conversation like I'd have with a friend and a lot different from what I was used to."

One of the characteristics of relationships on campus is that they are forged under extreme circumstances. As Jamie noted, "You rarely hang out together during the week. And on the weekends you go out and get drunk. The whole thing is so fake." She and Austin had the advantage of enjoying a whole summer together. She was lifeguarding every day; he would come to swim at the pool in the afternoons. They'd go out to a movie or for ice cream in the evenings. A day didn't go by when they didn't talk. He told her he admired her passion for school and her interest in politics. She loved hearing that; Jake, her former hookup buddy and an engineering major, had rarely praised her mind.

Normally back then, Jamie said, she would have pursued Austin. For some reason she didn't. But he pursued her, persistently. Three weeks into the relationship, Austin confessed that he was falling in love with her—and, as Jamie noticed, he was sober. That, too, was different.

"It was hard for me hear at the time," she recalled. "I didn't know what to say. I called my friends and said, 'Oh my God, this was supposed to be just a summer fling!' "

Two weeks later, after he told her again how much he loved her, she admitted she felt the same. "It was such a relief," she told me. "At Duke," she noted with a bit of exaggeration, "it would take two years to get to the point of saying that."

Austin, raised in a Christian home with conservative values, seemed more interested in getting to know her than getting her into bed. When they finally did have sex that summer, she discovered a depth of intimacy unlike any she had experienced. When she returned to school, she rented a contemporary one-bedroom apartment off campus and decorated it in colors of ocean blue and sunshine yellow. She framed his pictures and placed them alongside those of her family on her desk, her bookshelves and her bedside table. They continued to talk on the phone every day, and she sent him greeting cards with decorative stickers. They tried to visit each other at least once a month. When she felt stressed out over schoolwork, she'd take a phone break to talk to him and he would help her see how she could break down her assignments into manageable tasks. They dated through her sophomore and junior years.

"I know I have a million good qualities," she told me during that first interview at Duke early in her senior year, "but it is nice to have him tell me what they are. . . . God, the way he looks at me."

She thought back to freshman year and to the hookup partners she and her friends had—in her words—"settled for." "Every girl wants to be adored," she said. "If we had had what I have with Austin, we never would have done that." While I privately questioned her certainty, I couldn't help but notice how she beamed as she talked about Austin and be touched by it, given how long their relationship had lasted. "It doesn't get old and I love that," she said.

Austin was the perfect boyfriend: crazy about her and out of town, so he didn't interfere with her studies or her campus friendships. Only one shadow hung over their arrangement: the hookup habits of their respective campuses. On the weekends they were apart, they would go out drinking with friends. They both knew that scene—and each other's history.

Jamie said it was difficult for her to keep guys at arm's length. "They thought if I was talking to them, I'd go home with them." I heard this from lots of girls as the year progressed. In their mothers' generation, it would not have been the case. Guys assumed girls would not go to bed, especially if they had just met, though they might work hard to get them there.

Jamie also couldn't forget the number of girls Austin said had hit on him. "It still bothers me how much he slept with other girls before he met me, and I know my past bothers him," she said.

Insecurity comes with the territory of being in love. But in the hookup culture, it's not occasional, it's constant. "Neither of us would have done that stuff if we had known we were going to meet each other," Jamie said. I couldn't help but wonder if their phone calls to each other several times a day weren't partly an attempt to ease their anxiety.

In the summer before her senior year, Jamie accepted an internship on the West Coast, and Austin, who had graduated, accompanied her. He tried, and failed, to find a job, so she secured a volunteer assignment for him on the film set where she worked. They rented an apartment and shopped together for groceries. She cooked dinner; stir fry, made from ingredients picked up at a nearby Chinese market, was a favorite. They took day trips to the beach, visited museums, went out to eat and met lots of new people. "It was like living with a really good friend," she remembered.

Of all the girls I observed, she came the closest to finding a man who made her think about marriage. "The thought has crossed my mind," she confessed in early November.

By Austin's account, Jamie ran their relationship. Ever since her disastrous freshman year, when she was played by Jake, she was determined to have her boyfriend—and, more important, herself—under control at all times. She succeeded most of the time. But one incident she related suggested how easily that sense of control, and the confidence it bred, could disappear.

Late on one weekend night toward the end of her junior year, she and several girlfriends took a cab to Café Parizade, a swanky Mediterranean bar. They drank with other friends, danced a while, and before she knew it, it was one-thirty a.m. and last call at the bar. She searched for her friends and discovered they had all left, presumably with guys. Even one of her closest friends, who was traveling to Europe the next day and had sworn to see the night through with her, had vanished.

She had little choice but to walk outside and look for a taxi. There was none. Café Parizade, located in a modern brick building several miles from campus, is the only establishment in its neighborhood that is open on weekends, and is not a favorite stopping place for cabbies. Jamie started walking down a deserted street hoping to find a bus stop, drunk and scared at being out alone at such an hour. She dialed Austin on her cell phone and, when he answered, started crying. He calmed her down, told her to keep watching for a taxi and talking to him. Just then, a cab made a U-turn to pick her up.

What, I wondered, would she do if she lost Austin?

I would soon find out.

In early November, Jamie called to say that Austin had visited her at Duke for her twenty-first birthday and they had had "a little fight." He was working as a retail clerk in his hometown, and she thought he should be trying to get a better job. He'd say he was preparing his résumé but would never follow through. Despite his initial admiration for her interest in current events, he showed no interest in politics, a subject she loved to talk about. At her birthday dinner, they had had a few drinks and argued about his mother. She was beginning to question their long-term compatibility

So was he. Shortly after he returned home, during a telephone conversation, he uttered the immortal line, "I need some space."

"What are you saying?" she asked. Immediately her mind went to the only alternative she could think of. "You want us to be friends with benefits?" No, he said. He still loved her, and they were much more than friends.

He didn't really know what he wanted, he told me later, but he officially broke off the relationship over the phone in mid-December. The hardest part of that decision, she told me, "is that I had no choice in anything." The next three months—which, given that this was her senior year, could have been among her best at Duke—were hell.

I met her shortly after Christmas for lunch in Washington's upscale Georgetown neighborhood. It had been less than two weeks since Austin had dropped her, and more than a month since I had seen her. Looks-wise, she was still a match for any other young woman in the hamburger joint, but she had dropped a few pounds. Over the course of a couple of hours together, she picked at her fries and left most of a club sand-wich on her plate.

She told me that shortly before winter break, after Austin had al-legedly called it quits, he telephoned to say he looked forward to seeing her when she came home. He offered to pick her up at the airport that day and she accepted, thinking he had changed his mind about their re-lationship. He took her to his house, where, she said so softly I had to lean forward to hear her, they had sex. Afterward, he again expressed doubt about their future. She accused him of using her. He exploded.

"Never say that again," he told her.

Talking to me after their official breakup, Austin confessed to being as confused as Jamie's accounts made him sound. Having lived with her in Los Angeles over the summer and having made new friends in the fall, he was having second thoughts about how well they fit. He kept think-ing about little things that had happened in L.A.: the way she chastised him for spilling beer on her silk shirt, her insistence on keeping their apartment immaculate. Occasionally, he would drop a bit of pizza on the kitchen floor just to watch her reaction. "She knows what she wants and how to get what she wants. She definitely ran the relationship," he said.

He wasn't sure he wanted that. But he also thought she might be the classiest girl he'd ever meet. Thus the on-again, off-again behavior that characterizes so many relationships among young people this age—and makes young women reluctant to enter into anything more serious than a hookup.

Once Jamie returned to Duke after Christmas break, Austin contin-ued to call her. Jamie noticed, however, that when he was at work, he had stepped outside or into the bathroom. In college, he hadn't hesitated to chat when his buddies were around. Her radar went on alert. Maybe he was interested in someone else and didn't want his new friend to know he was still seeing her. She heard through a mutual acquaintance that he was hanging out with a coworker. But when she questioned him, he was always circumspect in his answers, saying that he and the young woman were "just friends." In the hookup culture, as she had painfully learned three years earlier with Jake, that could mean just about anything.

Austin's long-held worries about her continued as well. He'd phone at night and ask her where she was and if she was hooking up with anyone. That was how she had gotten over Jake, but this time, she thought, it wasn't the right strategy. She really didn't believe Austin was giving her up for good, and she kept telling herself that she could make their relationship work. He would occasionally say things that gave her hope. During one talk, he told her he had dreamed that she had sex with someone else and that when he woke up he realized that "I still want to spend my life with you."

Would a guy say that if he didn't mean it? she asked herself.

Yes, said her girlfriends and a favorite guy friend, all of whom she was calling several times a day. Drop Austin and block his calls, they advised. She didn't. Her mom gave her the same advice, even offered to pay any fee that might come with the call-blocking. She declined, and returned to school in January in a deep funk. On more days than not, she'd think, I've not only lost my boyfriend, I've lost my best friend.

On a Sunday morning in February, one day before Valentine's Day, Jamie ushered me into her apartment in Durham. Midmorning sunlight streamed through sliding glass doors onto a kitchen that was spotless and free of clutter. Four white kitchen chairs had been carefully pushed underneath the white table. She was, uncharacteristically, still in her pajamas and robe.

Pictures of her and Austin, along with ticket stubs and greeting cards, filled a pink "Austin box" sitting on a bookcase in her bedroom. Two children's books that he had purchased and inscribed were there as well. A pillow from him, white with blue lettering, lay on her bed, precisely in the center, between two other pillows. The embroidered inscription, from a Winnie-the-Pooh book, read, "If you live to be a hundred, I want to live to be a hundred minus one day, so I never have to live without you." It was evident that she really loved him and that he loved, or had loved, her.

A few days earlier, she had discovered that he was taking a vacation with his coworker. Nonetheless, a day before I visited her apartment, she had mailed him a Valentine's Day card. The day after I left, she received a card from him.

"I have never faced a situation where I didn't know what to do to arrive at a solution," she told me. "Even when I was hooking up before, part of me knew it was the wrong thing to do.

"If I stop calling him, he'll be with her. And if I continue to call, he'll go back and forth and just prolong it."

Though more mature than three and a half years earlier, at the moment she didn't feel much different than she had as that freshman waiting on a concrete bench for the bus to Jake's dorm. The control she had thought she possessed in her relationship with Austin was gone; she realized that he was defining what she did and how she felt.

"Austin knows if he wants to talk to me I'll pick up my phone, and that sucks," she said that day.

BACK ON HER TERMS

Time can be a healer, especially if your mother is in your corner. Jamie's mom, Ann, was so concerned about her daughter that she took her to the Caribbean island of St. John's over spring break. Jamie met a man there, a couple of years older than she, who, as she e-mailed me, was "mature, brilliant, funny" and "gorgeous . . . like Brad Pitt." He was a Yale graduate and taking some time off to work in the bar where they met. They talked on a couple of occasions but didn't do anything else because, she said, he had a girlfriend. It was just enough, however, to make her think she was finally getting over Austin. She returned to school with a month and a half to go and found herself wanting to put on makeup again and wear pretty skirts.

A freshman named Tyler who worked with her in an office on campus had been flirting with her on and off during the year. She hadn't paid a lot of attention, but now she was ready to flirt back. Within a couple of weeks, they were eating lunch together and Tyler was visiting her apartment. "He thinks everything I say is cute or funny!" she told me over the phone, sounding like a young girl describing a middle school crush.

Since most social activity took place with the upperclassmen on West Campus, Jamie found herself riding back and forth with Tyler on the bus between West and East Campus where Tyler, as a freshman, lived. It did not escape her that she was showing him the good manners that, almost four years earlier, Jake had not accorded her.

She was gaining enough distance from her relationship with Austin to realize it had taught her some things about what she wanted in a man. He should be intellectual, have attended good schools and know how to treat her well. It would help if he were good-looking, had money and were someone whom, as her mother put it, she "couldn't keep her hands off of."

Tyler fit the bill. But she was far from besotted over him, and it wasn't only the age difference. She was about to graduate and return to Los Angeles, where she hoped to work again in films. She needed to start a career unencumbered, so she laid out her rules to Tyler. Number one, he was to call her on his cell phone, not text-message her. Number two, he, not she, should do the calling. Number three, she didn't flirt in e-mails

or in instant messages. That's what telephones and face-to-face conversations were for.

Tyler belonged to one of the popular fraternities on campus, and she
suspected he had hooked up with a number of girls before. So here was
another nonnegotiable. "I don't do hookups," she told him. It was unlikely they would continue the relationship after graduation, she added.

It would have been easy for Jamie, once she started having problems
with Austin, to slip back into the unhooked social life she had known during her freshman year. Many of her friends, seniors like her, were still
bouncing from bed to bed. Hooking up was their way of playing at romance while controlling the unruly emotions that come with real romance. With so many things on their plates, so many things they wanted
to accomplish, that sense of control was crucial.

But Jamie was smart enough to have figured out that as powerless as
she felt with Austin, hooking up might have made her feel even more feeble. What she wanted was what she had had with Austin for most of
their two-plus years: a man who adored her day in, day out, and a loving relationship that empowered, rather than de-powered, her. Her
mother had been telling her this for several years—a mother's or father's voice can be crucial, as we'll see in the next section—and in the
end, she had to say, Mom had been right.

Tyler agreed to everything she asked and sought out time to be with
her. He'd walk her to class, holding her hand. He'd take her to a local
Asian restaurant where she loved the noodle bowls. He'd visit her apartment, where they'd watch a movie or Conan O'Brien and make out. "Is
this okay?" he would ask. "Is that?" He'd stroke her face and say,
"You're so beautiful. Do you know that?" In the week leading up to
graduation, he told he was in love with her.

"I'm having the time of my life right now," she told me. "I see all this stuff I've missed. It's so comfortable to be with someone who cares about you so much."

This was the Jamie who had approached me in class the previous fall, the Jamie who struggled valiantly, and would continue to struggle, to defy her culture and make love work on her terms. Some girls flee from the Tylers of the world, thinking they'll get in the way of who those girls want to be. Other girls embrace the Tylers as supporters of who they know they are. Jamie was one of the latter.

"Tyler knows I'm going to call the shots," she told me. That semester, her grade point average was the best in her four years at Duke: a 3.9 out of 4.

What It Looks Like,
What It Feels Like

A s they begin to engage the opposite sex seriously, girls are pretty sure they know what they want, and they feel entitled to it. Whether they're looking to hook up serially with anybody who appeals to them or, less often, for a more substantial relationship, what they want most, as Jamie illustrated, is control: They want to decide who, when and, above all, what happens between them and their partners, sexually and otherwise. In that sense, the same competitive instincts that young women bring to academics and sports apply equally to their social lives.

The nature of the contest changes as girls get older. In high school, they compete with other girls for the hot boys. They are motivated largely by status—winning admiration from their classmates for landing the most popular boys or boasting the longest list of conquests. In college, however, they come to see the boys as worthy sparring partners, and their girlfriends not as another battle front but as allies in an all-out war between the sexes. The prize from high school on is the feeling of power they get from setting their sights on a boy, seducing him and walking away at will, the better to avoid commitment, distractions and being hurt.

Tradition tells us that this is male behavior. We think of Casanova, James Bond or Sean Penn. Young women are saying it's their turn. In both high school and college, the hallmark of hooking up is that the boy, once recruited, is disposable. They may decide not to walk but take pride in the idea that they can. There's no such thing as cultivating the relationship. There's only the next game. This traditionally male social scheme has been reconstructed by girls who took a good look around and decided that it was better to be predator than prey, better do unto others before they do unto you. The fatal flaw in this scheme is that when girls believe this, they lose their bearings when the tables are turned. Some girls are surprised by the emptiness they feel when there's literally nobody new left to hook up with. Some are surprised when they discover that, having gotten sex, they want love, and they're unsure how to find it or, if they find it, how to handle it. Some are bewildered when the boy says he wants more than sex, or when he does the walking away. Hooking up leaves them unable to navigate in a world where their wants aren't the only consideration. That is, they don't know how to lose—and they don't know that even winning isn't a one-way street.

How would they know about losing, after all, when they're making up the rules as they go along?

High School

STORIES OF SIENNA, ANNA AND MIEKA

"I'm very competitive when it comes to both sports and boys.
When I'm in the middle of a good game, I'm confident, focused and
competitive. . . . I get this same sort of attention from boys when
I win them over, and from friends who are either jealous or
supportive of my relationships."
—SIENNA, FIFTEEN

It's hard to miss the starting forward on the field hockey team of one
of Washington, D.C.'s most prestigious private schools. Five feet,
four inches of tenth-grade muscle, she dribbles down the playing field
like a heat-seeking missile, her blond ponytail sailing behind her. When
she hits the ball, she hits hard. Her name is Sienna. She plays hockey and
soccer and boys, not necessarily in that order.

She came into my life online, taking issue with a newspaper article I
had written about "players," another term for teenaged bad boys. "Your
article made it seem that girls are helpless, lovesick Ophelias at the whim
of men who objectify and play them," she said. "What you failed to acknowledge is that girls are capable of the same cruel behavior, and possess the power to be players and break hearts, too.

"A new revolution of women is emerging," she continued. "Girls
are retaliating against the boys who once played them by using them. I
know several girls who pride themselves on being 'lady pimps,' claim-
ing to have no emotional attachment to guys, going out with multiple

boys at one time and manipulating them for their own benefit. Fellow girlfriends approve of this behavior and encourage each other."

She compared her two favorite hobbies. "I'm very competitive when it comes to both sports and boys. When I'm in the middle of a good game, I'm confident, focused and competitive. The better I play and the more goals I score, the more self-assurance and determination I gain. I constantly feel the need to outshine fellow teammates, not to mention pummel opposing teams. I love the praise I get after carrying my team to victory. I get this same sort of attention from boys when I win them over, and from friends who are either jealous or supportive of my relationships." Off the playing field, the goal, she wrote, "is all about getting/hooking up with the hottest, most well-known guys, and girls will spend a lot of time strategizing and manipulating their way into getting those guys."

My first interview took place in her comfortable family room in an upper-class Washington suburb, where tall windows gave onto a backyard of dark greens and dusky golds and bathed us in the light of a late-summer afternoon. Her mother, Beth, a fair-haired, trim figure in pastel cropped pants and a sleeveless blouse, had prepared herbal tea and a plate of sweets and sat in an armchair across the coffee table from me. Sienna, in low-rider jeans and a white knit top that showed off her evenly tanned complexion, sank easily into a couch nearby. After a few minutes of small talk, I asked her to explain what hooking up meant to her and her friends. She pulled no punches.

"Well, first you give a guy head," she said casually, "and then you decide if you like him and he decides if he likes you."

Beth, who had heard this explanation before, looked me straight in the eyes. "Can you believe this?" she asked softly. She picked up the plate on the coffee table. "Would you like a cookie?" Shortly after that, she excused herself so that Sienna and I could talk privately.

Over the next two hours, Sienna described a hookup culture much more rough-and-tumble than what I would learn about Duke from Jamie a month later. Or maybe it just seemed so when I thought of the tender ages of those taking part: fourteen, fifteen, sixteen and seventeen rather than eighteen, nineteen, twenty and twenty-one. Intercourse didn't happen frequently among Sienna's friends, at least until senior year of high school, but oral sex was no big deal. And the exchange of partners, if even half the number of what she described, was astounding.

She told of a couple of arrangements:

"Two of my friends are just friends and they hooked up. Really casual. Neither of them liked the other. That's so common now. It's nice for them because they don't have to worry."

Worry about what? I asked.

"Oh, you know, getting feelings for each other. You're drunk, or horny, the guy wants some, the girl wants some, and you won't have to worry about hurt feelings."

Sometimes, she said, relationships shrink to ordinary hookups. "I have a friend who broke up with her boyfriend and they're friends with benefits. They don't want a relationship." At other times, a relationship may consist only of regular hookups in the eyes of one partner, but mean something more to the other person, who must decide whether "a hookup relationship is better than no relationship at all."

She knew a girl who had decided recently to be satisfied with a hookup relationship. In Sienna's view, this was a wise choice. "At our age, we're supposed to be having fun," she argued. "There are too many hot guys and not enough time. That's what hooking up is all about."

Like the college women I would talk to later, Sienna and her friends were under a lot of pressure to "do it all": to make all A's (which required two to three hours of homework a night), play varsity sports year-round (which required traveling on weekends) and take part in community service or work at a paying job. Commitment to a boyfriend, carried out with the same intensity, seemed like one expectation too much. It's one thing, I thought, for older adult women to seek perfection in their jobs, childraising and housecleaning. It's something else again for fifteen-year-olds to already be victims of what Judith Warner calls, in her book about motherhood, "Perfect Madness." As I listened to Sienna that day, and later to other girls, I couldn't help but wonder whether any of them had had a real childhood.

One thing I had admired about Sienna from her first e-mail was the detailed, almost clinical way she described her social life and that of her friends. She was an astute observer of human behavior for someone so young, and admitted in one of our early conversations that she toyed with the idea of becoming a psychologist. I also noticed that she appeared to be as honest about herself as she was about her classmates.

There was a reason for that: She had had a lot of time on her hands to search her soul. Beth filled me in on the details after Sienna departed that afternoon.

A month earlier, while on the family computer, Beth had come across an e-mail Sienna had written to a friend about a boy named Justin with whom she was hooking up, drinking and occasionally smoking pot. That message, and the several days of tearful, occasionally fiery conversations that followed, told Beth that her oldest child was taking more risks on a weekly basis than Beth had taken in high school and college put together.

Beth had grown up in the Deep South, a blonde with a movie-star face, raised by parents who ruled with a firm hand and emphasized family reputation. She dated the same boy in high school for two years and still blushes at the memory of their first kiss. She graduated from college, went into business, met and married her husband, an attorney, at age twenty-five. Shortly after Sienna's youngest sibling was born, she stopped working to run the home and raise her kids—a job she took very seriously.

"Good grief," she said to her daughter after the e-mail discovery, "how can you do all of this at the same time!"

What astonished Beth in particular, she said during our first interview, was the number of school friends who Sienna said were more active than she was. Three of Sienna's best friends, one fifteen, the other two sixteen, had lost their virginity a year earlier. Girls Sienna knew, with their parents' permission, were inviting boys to coed sleepovers. Allegedly, the guys and girls slept in separate rooms, but Beth was dismayed nonetheless. In addition, Beth and her husband thought oral sex was something only a few girls did. Sienna told them otherwise and noted, "I delayed it at least a year from when everyone else started."

Reality may not have been as dire as Sienna suggested—teens tend to think their classmates are more daring than they actually are—but in Beth's view, it was plenty bad. She experienced that feeling, so common among parents these days, of being completely overwhelmed. No matter how much she thought she was on top of what her daughter was doing—and she spent a lot of time as a volunteer in school and on the phone with other parents, trying to stay on top—Sienna was clearly two or three steps ahead.

The irony did not escape her: She and her husband had decided on private schools for Sienna in part to reduce the chances of her taking such risks. They knew that friends and classmates influence kids' choices, but they hadn't realized just how much. They felt severely outflanked by a bunch of fifteen-, sixteen- and seventeen-year-olds. "Now they go from zero to ninety miles per hour in a heartbeat," Beth said.

Beth had taken her children to church, even as they moved into high school, determined to teach them the values she had learned. She had tried to be both diligent and fair with them. You can go out with friends, she told Sienna, but always let me know where you are. If you're sleeping over at a friend's house, I will call the parents in advance. She talked to Sienna about drinking, sex and love in general terms, assuming that there would be time to get more specific as her daughter faced each new challenge.

Should she have been more prescriptive in her rule-setting? Should she have made Sienna more responsible for chores around the house in the hopes of instilling in her a keener sense of personal responsibility? Her answer to both questions, looking back months later, was yes.

The randomness of hooking up, even without intercourse, especially bothered her. "What happens to the self when you are having sex indiscriminately?" she wondered aloud during a conversation several weeks after our initial meeting. "Sex should be something that happens after you feel connected to someone on an emotional level, a natural outgrowth of a relationship. I'd hate to see sex become so unimportant."

She grounded her daughter after the e-mail episode, feeling both afraid and sad. Normally, when advising Sienna, she rarely drew upon her own southern upbringing as a proper lady, knowing how dramatically manners and social mores have changed. But on this occasion she raised the idea of family honor. "There are certain things that are common," she told Sienna. "You don't want to be common."

From her first day of first grade, Sienna worried what other kids thought of her. "See how fat and ugly I was?" she asked one afternoon, showing me a tiny scrapbook photograph of a pretty girl with cascading curls. Beth remembers that third grade was particularly difficult for her daughter. The other girls formed an "I Hate Sienna Club," and Beth knew how hard that was on a child, particularly a girl. "We all want to be the one everyone loves," she said.

By sixth grade, however, the boys started noticing Sienna, and she quickly learned that if boys hung around, girls did, too. Coed groups became the social life form and remained so through high school. This enabled boys and girls to enjoy each other as friends. But it also meant that acceptable behavior was defined by the group. If most of the kids in your crowd were pairing up, you'd be looking for a steady boyfriend, too. If most of them were hooking up, the pressure to follow suit was equally intense. Some science even suggests that peer approval, more than puberty, defines when—and how—young people become sexually involved.

Sienna started practicing her game for real in seventh grade. "I got sick of having one boyfriend so I'd have two, one in school and one outside," she said. "I kept a list of boys to go out with next." At that age, she and her boyfriends didn't do much except hang out at lunch or after school, sneaking an occasional kiss. But other girls were in awe of her skills. She remembers one admirer in particular, named Abby, one of the most popular girls in seventh grade.

"I've been talking with the other girls," Abby told Sienna, "and we've decided you're the prettiest girl in our grade." Winning the boyfriend contest apparently meant winning the beauty contest, too. Playing guys got you the respect girls in middle school crave most: that of other girls.

Once she moved into high school, her game improved. A senior on the boys' basketball team started sending her instant messages, and pretty soon other seniors were doing the same. In the winter of freshman year, she attended what she called her "first real high school party," meaning a party where liquor was served. Alcohol was the guest of honor at virtually every party she went to after that, and weekends started on "Thirsty Thursday" night, just as they do at Duke and other colleges. Hearing Sienna's stories over the year, I realized that it is in high school where the notion takes hold that if you're going to drink, you might as well get drunk—like if you're going to hook up, you might as well hook up with several partners. The idea of moderation in either drinking or sex is, for some students, a foreign concept.

Sienna was not one of those students. But several of her friends were. She remembers two things in particular about that "first real party": Several older girls tried unsuccessfully to pour liquor down her throat, and she met Justin. A tall, athletic, shaggy-haired boy from public school,

Justin exhibited what she called "a bad-ass attitude" and paid no attention to her despite her efforts to flirt with him that night. She remembers thinking, I can break him.

She did, but only sort of. He would call her, but not when he said he would. He'd stop by her house, but not necessarily when she invited him. When they were together, though, "we could talk about everything that bothered us." The physical chemistry they shared was intense. As a bonus, the fact that he didn't belong to her private school crowd freed her to hang out with other guys when she wasn't with him. Attitudes are different now than they were in her mother's day, she told me. Then, a girl was considered no-account if she cheated on a steady boyfriend. Not anymore.

In May of freshman year, at a school dance, Sienna met Adam, a junior from another private school. She went to a movie with him, invited him over to her house and kept track of him and Justin—and a sophomore named Chad, with whom she had a short fling—in a journal. In both high school and college, girls describe three kinds of sexual relationships, and Sienna was juggling all three: Chad, the one-night stand; Adam, the casual, occasional hookup; and Justin, the boyfriend. Physical intimacy with Justin was limited until late May, when they engaged in reciprocal oral sex. She extended the same privilege to Adam the same weekend, then had second thoughts about whether that had been a wise move.

"Wow, that was pretty retarded," she recalled saying to herself on Adam's night.

But it gave her a chance to impress Adam, who was older, and a chance to impress her friends, most of whom she believed to be ahead of her sexually. Two guys in two days? Wow.

"You want to be able to say, 'I have done it, too,' to feel old and mature, part of the group. Nobody likes someone who's uptight."

She didn't lose any sleep over cheating on Justin because she figured he was cheating on her, too. To be faithful, and to give up the opportunities to be a player, would, she wrote me, "make me feel weak, used, and sort of like the pathetic stereotype of a woman in the relationship. I'd much rather feel empowered and strong and even manipulative." By the end of her freshman year, Sienna felt she had arrived. "One guy told me I am one of the top five hottest girls in high school. I might suck at school. [She didn't.] But I'm hot."

She didn't worry at this point about contracting a disease. She had heard the warnings in sex education: Herpes, syphilis, gonorrhea, hepatitis and the human papillomavirus (linked to cervical cancer) could be transmitted through oral sex. But infection seemed too remote a possibility to stop using what she had to win over boys of her choice, and neither she nor the girls she knew ever used condoms or dental dams during oral sex. It was only after Beth, upon discovering the ill-fated e-mail message, took her to a gynecologist to be tested for disease that Sienna began to rethink the pace of her behavior.

Mouth and tongue are two of the most powerful weapons in the sexual skirmishes of high school and college. According to national data released in mid-2005, one out of two teenagers between fifteen and nineteen has given or received oral sex. In the CDC sample, teens from white, middle- and upper-income families like Sienna's were more likely to have engaged in oral sex than other groups. Earlier surveys of such scope don't exist, so there's no way to know how this compares to past generations of teens. But adults in their forties and older, when they hear about how common oral sex has become, believe that it occurs more frequently now than when they were young and are particularly struck by young people's blasé attitude about it. Bill Albert, a middle-aged communications director for a teen pregnancy prevention organization, put it this way: "We used to talk about sex in terms of first base, second base and so on. Oral sex stayed in the dugout. Now it's in the on-deck circle."

. . .

Like many teenaged girls, Sienna talked endlessly about boys, so much
so that it would have been easy to assume that her entire week, and that
of her girlfriends, was consumed with them. That was not the case. In
fact, Friday and Saturday nights were usually the only times Sienna hung
out with Justin. Early sophomore year, she admitted to me that she was
getting bored with him. During the week, deprived of phone privileges,
she had to resort to the computer to carry their relationship forward.
Her lively voice, vivid gestures and flirtatious eyes had given way to
smiley faces and words in all caps. Without the spontaneity and im-
provisation required during conversations on the phone or face-to-face,
she found it harder to express herself or get excited by him.

"We've typed 'I like you' so much it's beginning to get tiresome," she
said, the weariness in her voice unmistakable.

Workplace experts have remarked that young people don't express
themselves as clearly as previous generations did. Part of the reason,
they suggest, is that youth don't listen well. With e-mails and instant
messages, they don't have to; they can read and re-read something they
receive; there's no need for an immediate, spontaneous response. Sienna's remarks suggest that poor communication skills can be found in
relationships as well. When Justin came over to her house to hang out,
they'd watch TV and not talk for long stretches of time. "I thought
maybe after you went out for a while that's all you did," she told me. I
was reminded immediately of Jamie, the Duke freshman, who had complained about spending hours in front of the TV with Jake at his fraternity house. If this was what passed for good times in a relationship, no
wonder they got bored.

Dating conventions of several decades ago assumed that a young
man would think up new activities to keep his love interest interested.
Such considerations are not necessary in a hookup culture where one

partner can easily be traded for another. Without having previously experienced the thoughtfulness of decent boyfriends, many girls, sadly, have no idea what they should expect.

Less than a month after our initial interview, and nine months into their relationship, Sienna broke up with Justin. Beth had tried to convince her to give Justin more time. At least it was a relationship, Beth said to her daughter, and it could be worked on. What Beth didn't know, Sienna told me, was that Justin was pressing her to go "all the way," and in their culture, she was finding fewer reasons to say no.

Justin was ready to split up, and they parted amicably. That was important to Sienna for two reasons. The first had to do with keeping up her connections with friends from his school. In just a few years she had gone from having no friends to lots of friends, and she was proud of that. "Never burn your bridges," she'd say. The second reason followed the first: Her friends would judge her on how well she pulled off the split—and how quickly she got back into the game.

Fortunately for her, the fall social schedule was revving up, which meant a party at someone's house almost every weekend. She would have liked to give parties at her house but didn't, fearing how some of her classmates might act and her mother's eagle eye. Fortunately, her friends threw parties. One was a birthday celebration for a sophomore girl held on the grounds of the family's large lake house. Dozens of other sophomores showed up, some carrying water bottles filled with liquor and some with marijuana in their pockets. A few kids danced, but the majority of guests spent most of their time hooking up.

"Some people, once they got drunk, hooked up in front of everyone," she said, "including some girls who guys asked to kiss in front of them. Some people snuck into the woods, and a couple of couples went down the hill. There were only two real couples there, so for the most part it was friends hooking up randomly with friends." The girl's parents, patrolling the party, would split up partners, "but eventually the couples

ended up just going back and doing it again," Sienna said. They also exchanged partners since hooking up, absent strong feeling, can get pretty
monotonous over the course of an evening. "Most of us hooked up with
at least two people," she said. Until then, their activities had sounded like
what would have been called, a couple of generations ago, necking and
petting. The freewheeling partner exchange, however, was a new twist.

At another party that fall, several of Sienna's girlfriends, drunk and
once again bored, cornered a freshman girl, took off her blouse and bra
and pushed her into a bathroom with a boy. Sienna wasn't sure what
happened after that, but she was dismayed. "I don't know what would
have happened if there had been more time, better places, fewer chap-
erones," she said.

After that second party, Sienna came home and collapsed on her bed,
crying. She had limited herself to soft drinks and water that evening because as the proud new owner of a driver's license, she had driven herself to the party. Like anyone who has been the only sober one in a crowd,
she discovered how foolish, even mean, drunks can be. "I saw way too
much," she told me.

The party would be the talk of school on Monday—something of a
coup for those who attended. But Sienna and her friends were smart
girls, and the possible implications of their wild behavior didn't escape
them. In the days following the party, they discussed in e-mails and instant messages whether they were becoming alcoholics and wondered
why they sometimes treated each other badly.

"What the hell is going on with us?" they asked each other, and
"What is our problem?" Sienna was beginning to worry that her grades
were suffering. "While all this is happening it's fun," Sienna told me.
"The next day it sucks, and the day after that it's, When are we going to
do it again?"

Having attended her school since kindergarten, she knew her several
hundred classmates in grades nine through twelve pretty well and could

only think of four honest-to-goodness couples in that group. Everyone else, if they paired off at all, hooked up. "I have one friend who hasn't hooked up," Sienna said. "She really wants to, but she doesn't have game."

In an odd way, hooking up at parties was keeping them connected. They'd say things like "I gave John head, then he hooked up with Cassie who hooked up with Brett who hooked up with me." Theirs was not simply the behavior of a handful of spoiled, rich kids. In one eighteen-month study, James Moody, a sociology professor at Ohio State University, found similar connections when he mapped the sexual relationships of a largely white public high school in the Midwest. He expected to find a core of sexually active students with a few branches. Instead, he found long chains of associations including one that tied together 288 of approximately 1,000 students in the school. His diagram resembled a necklace with assorted clusters of baubles attached—a student in one circle being intimate with a student in another circle and so on. This, he said, had serious health implications.

It's safe to say that Sienna and her classmates would not have carried on individually as they did in a group. Had one of them been brave enough on those two nights to try to stop the more risqué behavior, others might have stepped in to assist. But each was waiting for someone else, and as a result no one did.

"The only people telling me not to do this stuff are my parents," Sienna said. I wondered at the time, Would Beth and her husband be enough to keep her out of trouble for the rest of the year?

In early winter of her sophomore year, Sienna started hooking up with a senior at her school named Mark. He came to her on the rebound from one of her classmates but she didn't mind. By her friends' standards, he was a catch. She thought he was hooking up only with her but a few weeks after they started seeing each other, she heard rumors at school that he was having sex with his old hookup partner. When she asked them, both denied it. But she found a message from the girl to Mark that seemed to confirm what she had heard, and she stopped speaking to Mark for two weeks.

Her anger surprised her. She knew hookups weren't necessarily exclusive, even if they lasted weeks. That's one of their biggest attractions. As she put it, "Even if you get jealous, you can't tell someone what to do and he can't tell you what to do." Was she mad because he appeared to have seized the upper hand? Had lied to her? Was using her? As Beth would observe later, "When love equals sport, it's hard to sort these things out, especially when you're sixteen."

The drama of her social life began to take its toll on her interest in school and her grades. "I'm having trouble caring about school," she said in an interview in her family room, five months after my first visit. "I see no reason why I should know when the Roman empire collapsed." She received her first C as a grade for the winter quarter, prompting warnings from her parents that she couldn't make another one if she wanted to be accepted into a Division I university. As someone who enjoyed being regarded as playing at the top of her game in everything, she feared her status was slipping. "People used to say I was a really good student," she said. "I used to be a lot smarter than people, now I'm dumber."

Eventually, when convinced by both her friends that what they had was over, she started seeing Mark again. Late in the winter, the two of them compiled a list of all the places they could hook up and started knocking places off the list: an elevator, the snow, a hospital parking lot. She didn't call Mark her boyfriend; girls rarely call such friends boyfriends. But he did hold the title of being, as she put it, "the second person (after Justin) I don't mind spending a lot of time with." So she started to worry when, in early spring, she picked up signs that his ardor was cooling. She mentioned this one night on the phone, and he admitted that she was right, but not because he was no longer interested in her. He was, in fact, more interested—in her thoughts, opinions and affection. He wanted more from her, including a promise of exclusivity.

"He thought all I wanted was to hook up. I thought that was what *he* wanted."

She couldn't imagine what they might do together as a couple since they mostly partied with friends. She could think of only one thing to say: "Well, maybe we can watch a movie tonight?"

Earlier in the year she had told me that once a girl convinces a boy to like her, she often gets bored. "Boys get needy," she said, "and clingy. They have to hang out with you all the time. My girlfriends and I call the feeling 'the yucks.' " Her observation gave me pause. Has the increasingly aggressive sexual behavior of young women prompted a change in young men as well? Is there something inherent in the mating dance that if one partner pursues and catches his or her conquest, the other partner automatically assumes the role of the pursued? Biology tells us that the male in many species pursues a female in order to produce an heir and, once he has impregnated the female, will attempt to leave her to find another female. The impregnated female, however, will try to keep the male by her side to help feed and shelter the new family. The female becomes, in effect, "clingy." Sienna's comment raised the possibility that when gender roles are switched, the same reactions may occur in reverse.

Was Mark giving her "the yucks"? I asked Sienna. Not exactly, she replied. "But now I feel like he wants to go for a walk in the park and hold hands. I don't know if I want to do that."

They had been hooking up for four months, including their short break, when they had this conversation about the nature of their relationship, initiated by him. And when they did talk, his interest panicked her. Another example of how gender roles are changing, I thought. Back in the 1970s and 1980s, a girl in her situation would probably have been the one to bring up the subject of an "us," and the guy might easily have taken a walk, fearing that she was getting too dependent.

Her hesitation to declare them a couple made some sense. True intimacy involves opening up to someone on a deeper level than other people are permitted to see. Sienna and Mark had disclosed very little about themselves to each other. They had been more focused on playing the hookup game skillfully than on getting to know each other. What a dilemma: They didn't want to reveal too much about themselves because they never knew when their relationship would end. But if they didn't share their likes and dislikes, and didn't show some vulnerability as well as strength, they wouldn't experience a real relationship.

Jamie could have told her this. But Jamie was eighteen when she met Austin, and certain that she could control that relationship. Sienna was sixteen, not as sure of her power, and more addicted to hookup behavior than Jamie ever was. As she put it, "When you're hooking up, you don't say 'I love you,' even if you think you might."

She saw no reason to get serious with Mark. He was headed for college in the fall, while she had two more years with the same crowd at the same school. She couldn't make any promises about what she would or would not do. At the same time, she worried about the next two years. She was still a virgin, and if her social life continued on the same course, the pressure to shed that label, already intense, would increase. Unlike in past generations, boys these days expected girls to "give it up" eventually, she said.

Near the end of the school year, Sienna and I met for Sunday brunch in a trendy café of polished red leather seats and lots of chrome. Over the course of the year she had grown an inch or two and her face had lost some of its baby softness to the more angular look of an older teenager. I asked her to look ahead to next year, her junior year, and then to college. But first she wanted to look back, and she made a remarkable confession for someone so young.

"I do have an addiction problem," she began. "I don't do hard-core drugs, and I don't drink during the week. But if I drink, I drink a lot. If I shop, I shop a lot. If I hook up, I hook up a lot. I can't go to a party one night and not go to a party the next night."

I was hearing from her what I had observed in other girls who, like Sienna, were smart and ambitious. Being the best at whatever they did was their way of winning admiration, affection and love. Their drive, well explained in Sienna's first e-mail, was so ingrained that slowing down at anything was difficult, even when they wanted to.

Earlier at brunch, she had said she told her mother that she felt like she "didn't have time to breathe," and that Beth had said she could quit one of her sports. "But what would I do with my time?" she responded.

Sienna might not have admitted it to her mother, but she did to me: Such conversations with Beth had been her anchor during the year. Beth knew her daughter listened to her friends—discovering the computer message early in the year told her how much—but she had hoped her voice, over time, would be the strongest. That's what every bit of research she had read told her, but given what had happened in Sienna's sophomore year, she wasn't sure.

She needn't have worried. Even during her grounding, Sienna had conceded to me that she understood her mom's reasoning. "I told her she is trying to encourage me to have good behavior." There was little doubt in my mind that Beth was the reason Sienna was still a virgin.

Beth had taken away Sienna's instant-messaging and e-mailing privileges early in the year and didn't restore them once Sienna was off restriction. "As a parent you have to look at what you can control," she told me. Sienna protested but still appreciated the fact that she had a mom who cared, unlike girls she could name.

"A lot of my friends are able to party all night, sleep over at each other's houses—boys and girls," she said. "They feel like their parents don't care. Their friends are their family."

Being with Mark had settled her down, she said. He was less inclined to drink than her past partners and, in fact, the two of them didn't drink when they were together. "We had fun anyway," she said with a half-smile, adding, "I need someone who is a good influence."

She was under no illusions that simply because she was maturing, the next few years would be easier. In fact, she suspected they'd get harder.

"Watching what my friends in older grades are doing," she wrote in an e-mail, "by senior year some people will be experimenting with cocaine and other more serious drugs. Some will be having more sex and just continuing to drink and smoke weed. It takes more to excite and shock them. Also, a lot of upperclassmen think it's funny to 'adopt' underclassmen to corrupt and take them to parties to get them high and drunk and hook up with them."

In two more years, on whatever college campus she landed, she'd be wondering not what to do with her weekend but what to do with her entire week.

"I swear if college is worse, I don't know what the world is coming to."

"I wish it was like I hear it used to be. I think, Wouldn't it be nice if this guy I like liked me enough to ask me out? I hope that will happen before the end of high school. Or at least in college."—ANNA, FIFTEEN

I first met Anna, a tenth-grader at a public high school in Washington, D.C., at a Starbucks coffee shop on a busy avenue in northwest Washington. Slightly built, with light-brown hair that hung limply around her face, she was wearing the teenaged girl uniform: blue jeans and a camisole with spaghetti straps. Her divorced parents, both professionals, lived only a few streets away from each other, so she'd visit one for a while, then the other. She described them as "old-fashioned liberals," and said she enjoyed a good relationship with her mother. Right away, she wanted me to know that she wasn't a normal teenager because she hadn't hooked up very much. "My eighth-grade sister has more of a social life than I do," she said, smiling wanly.

There was a reason for that. She had had a horrid ninth-grade year in junior high, bouncing back and forth between parents, suffering from depression and distancing herself from friends. She had worn sloppy, boyish clothes to school, had talked about women's rights and been labeled a "feminazi" by some of her male classmates.

"I didn't give a shit who I was impressing," she recalled.

This year, she was enrolled in a public high school in northwest Washington with about 1,400 students, or more than three times the number of kids in Sienna's private school. The students were more diverse than Sienna's classmates: half African-American, with Hispanics and whites making up the rest and one-third eligible for reduced-cost or free school lunches. Anna moved easily among the different groups but put most of her effort into working her way back into her old crowd from junior high. She assumed the role of mother to some of her friends, accompanying them to parties and handing out condoms. Her own mother, more permissive than Sienna's mom, knew she did this, and trusted her not to go too far sexually herself. "Let me guess," she'd sigh as Anna left for a party, "there won't be any parents there."

Anna had begun to notice boys—really notice boys, as in "I'll come to school looking like crap, see a hot guy in the hallway and the next day think twice about what I wear." She paused, then added, "I don't say I'm doing it for the guys even though I partly am."

Kind of like hooking up with a boy to win his interest? I asked.

"Maybe. But I'm looking for a boyfriend, not a hookup partner."

This early in my reporting, I hadn't heard a girl say that, and in fact, over the coming year's countless discussions with different girls, I heard it from only one other. To this generation of girls, the word "boyfriend" suggested being tied down to someone—or worse, unable to function independently. Their interpretation made some sense to me; I remembered how, when I was their age, if my girlfriends and I didn't have boyfriends we thought there was something wrong with us. These girls didn't seem to labor under that assumption.

Where Sienna pursued hookup partners in order to feel acclaimed, Anna desired a boyfriend because she wanted romance in her life. She suspected the odds were slim; in her school she knew of only four recognizable couples. She believed that if she had any chance of finding such a guy, she would have to appear to be to playing by the same rules as everyone else so that boys would not think of her as a prude. That meant hanging out in the hallways with certain kids, going to parties and pretending to hook up occasionally, which, as the year progressed, she did with less and less pretense. Girls are sucked into the hookup culture for different reasons: Sienna's was to win status, Anna's to find love.

She had arrived that fall afternoon accompanied by a petite, dark-haired friend named Bianca. The two girls chose a small table near the door so they could keep an eye on a steady stream of customers. This particular Starbucks, around the corner from school, was their version of a 1950s malt shop. As intrigued as they were with the idea of talking to a reporter, they didn't want to miss any action.

We picked up lattes, and Bianca bought a package of mini-carrots to munch on.

How does hooking up start? I asked the girls as we took seats.

"You usually sort of like the guy," Anna said.

"Although it could be random," Bianca added.

How do you make your first move?

"If you see him in the hall, you pick up your chin, pull down your top and stick your butt out," Bianca said.

"If you're across from him in class," said Anna, "you cross your legs toward him instead of away from him. Or, you just ask him, 'Wanna hang out?' "

Where does the hooking up take place?

"A party at someone's house. Usually."

The word "usually" was significant. Unlike conventions of the past, rules of their unhooked culture varied from girl to girl, although all were designed for maximum freedom. In Anna's crowd, this meant that a girl wouldn't accompany a guy to a party unless she already was in a serious relationship with him. She would go instead with girlfriends, ideally in her own car if she had one, so that she could escape alone or with someone of her choosing at any time. She would try to find out in advance who was going to be there, who was already attached and who was fair game. Since competition could be fierce, she would rarely tell anyone whom she was going after.

"If you mention you think a guy is hot, your friend may be, 'Oh, he *is* hot. I'm gonna go get with him,' " Anna said.

Her friend Bianca nodded. "And you don't want sloppy seconds."

To listen to these girls, you'd think that they had it all figured out and that guys didn't stand a chance against them. Where Jamie wanted to control one guy at a time, they, like Sienna, wanted to assert their power over all of the guys.

"To say I did this because I wanted to is a lot better than saying I let him do it to me," said the still-feminist Anna.

"There's a guy I don't even like," she continued. "If I'm in a bad mood, I can be very cold toward him. The next day, if I even poke him in the back as a joke, he's like a little puppy dog. It's fun being in control like that. There are very few guys who, if you make a move, will say no."

Bianca nodded. "Hooking up," she said, punching the air with a carrot for emphasis, "is saying 'I can have you whenever I want you and I can have whoever I want.' "

Words that some girls use to describe the guys they're hooking up with carry this attitude of ownership. I've heard girls call guys "my toy," "my plaything," a "filler boy" (until the real thing comes along), even "my bitch." It's as if they think that by speaking as coarsely as guys sometimes do, they will be perceived as having as much power. And if such words are used on them, the words won't carry the same sting.

It's not just their language that differs dramatically in their everyday exchanges, according to longtime teachers Robert and Mary Louise Payne. Between them, the Paynes have taught Latin for forty-plus years to public-school children, Mary Louise at an urban school, and Robert in an upper-income Maryland suburb.

"We used to get onto kids for holding hands in school," says Mary Louise. "Then it was kissing. Now I see girls softly kneeing guys in the groin. I'd rather have the kissing."

Robert tells similar tales. "I'll be walking along the hallway and hear a girl tell another girl, 'We're going to his house after school and have sex.' We recently held a student assembly on sexually transmitted diseases. A girl stood up and asked how hot a hot tub could get before it would melt a condom."

For all their professed sense of control, however, both girls admitted harboring feelings of self-doubt. Anna explained:

"In school, a girl will ask herself, What did he mean when he said 'Hi' that way? Did he really call me for homework? Did he hold my hand a little longer than normal when he handed me that pencil?

"Or say a boy whom you party with on Saturday night e-mails you a message on Sunday afternoon. Does it mean he actually likes you? Wants to do something with you? You print it out, look at it and ask over and over, What does it mean? You can't come right out and ask him if you're make-out buddies or does he want you just as a friend."

Why?

"Because he might reject you."

Substitute the word "boyfriend" for "make-out buddy" and that conversation could easily have taken place when their mothers were dating. I had to ask myself, If girls battle the same insecurities their mothers did earlier, how much power have they really gained?

"When you hear someone you like has hooked up with someone else, your cheeks burn and you cry. You cared more than you realize," Bianca admitted that first afternoon. She said she had a particular boy in mind, but declined to elaborate.

No one likes being shut down, even confident girls. They'd much rather ditch a potential partner, as Anna did at a debate tournament at a local high school a few weeks after our first conversation. Her teammates had decided to play poker during a break in the competition and she didn't feel like playing. A boy named Jason from her school, whom she barely knew, asked her to take a walk with him outside. She agreed halfheartedly.

"I thought he wanted to just talk or something," she recalled.

They walked around the back of the school and Jason asked her, "Wanna hook up?"

"I'm not in the mood," she replied.

He asked her a second, then a third time, and finally she gave in.

"Fine, why not?"

They kissed and fondled each other for a while and then Jason said he wanted to go further. She declined but he pushed on. "I'm at the point of no return," he said.

"I'm going back now," she replied. She knew that if her mom, as a girl, had made out with someone she wasn't remotely interested in, that girl would have been called a tramp. Her mom had told her that, and she had told her mom that that wouldn't be the case now. Like Sienna, who hooked up with three guys over the same short period of time, she was enjoying the freedom of being unhooked not just from a partner but from the social expectations that, in her view, had hindered her mother.

That's not to say there were no expectations. When Anna returned to the tournament, a debate partner asked where she had been. She hesitated. An unspoken rule of the unhooked culture was you didn't hook up outside your clique—a carryover from past generations, perhaps, but also stemming from the possibility of acquiring a disease. Someone outside your circle of friends was more likely to carry an infection than someone you knew, or at least girls thought so, as evidenced by the number of times they'd tell me about a sexual encounter with a friend and say something like "I know him. He's clean. He'd never go out with a skank."

Anna, however, didn't want to lie to her debate partner.

"You're never going to believe it," she said. "I hooked up with Jason."

Her friend raised her eyebrows a bit, but said, "Well, thank God. I was afraid you were out there smoking."

Anna could now add her name to the list of girls who had hooked up for no good reason. And she might have to do it again at some point. "If you don't hook up, or only hook up once, *that's* considered weird," she said.

In early winter, Anna met me at the same Starbucks and brought along two new girls—Zoe, sixteen, a frizzy-haired, extremely shy young woman who was probably her best friend, and Jill, also sixteen, a brunette with big brown eyes and a big voice. Both had hookup experiences they could share, Anna told me privately. After running through my usual first questions, I steered the conversation to oral sex. In my generation, I began, kids, especially guys, talked about getting to first, second or third base with a partner or, on rare occasions, hitting a home run. What was their continuum, I asked in a low voice, looking around in the hope that none of the older adults nearby, reading or typing on laptops, could hear us.

In particular, I asked, when might a girl "go down on" a guy?

"I always heard about the four F's," Anna volunteered. "French [kiss], feel [up], finger, fuck."

"But oral sex has got to be in there somewhere," her friend Jill said.

The three of them put their heads together, whispered and counted on their fingers. "Got it!" Jill squealed. "For us it's feel, finger, fellatio, fuck! French kissing is so tame it doesn't count anymore." If the patrons sitting near us heard anything, and I can't see how they didn't, they had the good manners not to react.

For another hour, Anna and her friends dished about sex as nonchalantly as they might discuss their daily calorie intake or workout routines. Carmela, a fifteen-year-old classmate, joined the group briefly and revealed that she hadn't hooked up with anyone yet. She wasn't looking forward to doing it, she said, but she guessed she would sometime during the year. "Sex is just something you should experience, like drugs," she said.

Adults frequently ask me how I persuade young people to talk frankly about sex. The truth is, such frankness comes naturally to them, a by-product of the movies they watch, the music they listen to and the discussions they've had in sex education. Girls are remarkably candid with each other (some might say crude) on all issues relating to sex, and openly so, not whispering to each other behind cupped hands. One high school girl, recently back from field hockey camp, recalled a conversation she and several teammates had late one night in their cabin.

"How many fingers do you use to masturbate?" she said one girl asked.

"I use three," another camper answered.

"I've used a vibrating toothbrush," yet another girl said.

"Does anyone else shake when they touch their clit?" someone wanted to know.

The conversation turned to techniques of oral sex.

"How fast do you move your hand?" asked a girl.

"Do you spit or swallow?" asked another.

Such an exchange does not surprise Sandy French, a young communications professor who teaches public speaking at Pennsylvania State University. French allows her students to choose their speech topics several times a semester, and when they choose something on the subject of sexuality, which is not infrequently, "their language is all about technique, not intimate feelings or choices," she told me. "It's, What can I use to get you to want me?"

French said she doesn't want her daughter growing up with the inhibitions that can accompany staying silent about one's body and desires. But like Sienna's mother, she is bothered by the fact that girls' conversations take place anywhere, at any time, in front of almost anybody— and seem so detached from passion.

THE CRUSH

Locker-room lingo allows girls to put distance between what they're doing and how they feel about what they're doing. But it doesn't stop some of them from wanting more.

As the school year advanced, Anna developed a secret passion for a classmate named Noah. Noah was the mirror image of a young Patrick Swayze, ruggedly good-looking with straight brown hair and brown eyes that always made him appear as if he were thinking about something or someone far away. "Everyone has had a crush on him," Anna said.

She flirted with Noah in class. She fantasized about going on a date with him because her mother told her this would mean he was interested in her opinions as well as her body. She feared, however, that they might just hook up and if they did, "I wouldn't be sure what it meant, whether he liked me at all. In fact, if he asked me if I wanted to hook up, I'd be hurt. If it's someone you like, you usually don't ask." She had told her mother this, and her mom, who had recently started dating again after her divorce, had simply shaken her head. "If it was like that for me now, I'd go crazy," she'd told Anna.

Noah was already hooking up with another girl at school, so Anna figured she had no chance. But when she started rehearsals for a winter school play, she was delighted to learn that he was playing drums in the orchestra. After the last performance, each musician was given two roses, and Noah complained about having to carry them to the cast party.

"I'll carry them if you'll give them to me," Anna said. Noah immediately knelt down on one knee and handed them to her. They left the school together and, without saying anything, wandered away together in the opposite direction from the location of the party. They walked for ten or fifteen minutes, talking and pretending not to notice the route they had chosen. Then she finally said, "You know what? I think the party is back that way."

"Oh yeah," he said, and they turned around.

That incident, as innocent as it was, occupied Anna's thoughts for several weeks. This, I realized, was what we used to call puppy love, what girls today call a crush. Some girls are able to suppress it, but others can't. It was easy for us to admit to our girlfriends when we had such crushes because love was valued in our culture. It's not so easy for girls today. Anna kept her feelings about Noah to herself.

Winter break intervened, and Anna left on a family trip to Nicaragua. She brought along her friend Zoe, and one night they hung out at a bar with two Nicaraguans: José, a seventeen-year-old whom Zoe knew, and

José's friend Daniel, eighteen. Right away the girls noticed something un-usual about these two young men: "They opened doors for us and pulled out our chairs at the bar," Anna recalled.

Daniel's father was a wealthy inventor and owned a large home with a swimming pool just outside Managua. Daniel took his friends back to the house, and he and Anna slipped away to a dark, empty room, where they talked and made out, though only a little by American standards. "I was a little tipsy," she admitted. "In the U.S., you can't have a conversa-tion with a guy alone in your underwear in the dark. But we did. We talked a couple of hours, just the two of us. We had a surprising amount in common. You'd think an eighteen-year-old would take advantage of a fifteen-year-old, but he didn't."

"We hooked up, but I started it. He let me lead. If I had asked to go to his bedroom, he would have. But I didn't. It was really fun."

Daniel had clearly inspired her, and by the time she returned to Wash-ington, still marveling over the night in Managua, she had talked herself out of Noah. "He was a right-brain thing," she said.

New Year's Eve produced more excitement. Anna accompanied Zoe to a party of mostly college-aged kids where, Anna said, "Everybody was smashed, hooking up and having sex." Anna was approached by a cute guy with an Iggy Pop haircut. "His name was Michael, I think." They talked for a few minutes and then Michael asked her to go upstairs with him. A little mutual making out, like she had done with Daniel, couldn't hurt, she thought. As Michael led her upstairs, she passed Zoe coming down the stairs with a guy. Zoe leaned over to her, laughing, and whis-pered, "He just wants you to suck his cock."

Forewarned, Anna walked into a bedroom with Michael and told him right away, "I'm not having sex with you, and I'm not sucking your cock." Michael turned on his heels and walked out of the room. Later that night, Zoe confessed to Anna that she had hooked up with two guests at the party and that Michael had been one of them. Anna got upset, not out of jealousy but out of concern for her friend. She had counseled Zoe in the past against going further with partners than she wanted to. Michael had used Zoe and Zoe obviously knew that, given what she had whispered to Anna on the stairs. What was happening to Zoe's self-esteem?

Winter break produced one hopeful story, in Anna's eyes. It involved Maria, Anna's "best, best friend" from the previous summer. Maria, who had never even kissed a boy, had met a guy a year older than she at summer camp. They fell in love, and when she returned to Washington and he to Oregon, they wrote long e-mails to each other every day. Anna learned that Maria had flown to Oregon to spend a week with her boyfriend and his family. While she was there, they had made love several times.

"How incredible is that?" Anna asked me. "She had her first kiss and lost her virginity to the same boy. She told me it was amazing."

Now the couple was continuing to write and considered themselves in a relationship, according to Anna, "although they know it can't be exclusive."

As her sophomore year sped by, Anna got over her reluctance to approach guys directly for affection. She was trying to combine the two sides of her personality, she said. Her feminine side, honed over the year I knew her, was telling her, "Admit it, you like boys, and you like looking attractive in order to catch their eye." The feminist side, developed the year before in ninth grade, was conceding, "Okay, go for it. Hook up if you want to in a pretty short skirt and makeup. But don't play silly games. Take charge, and keep the upper hand."

"I'm more sexual," she told me in our last interview, alone, at Starbucks. "If there's someone I want to hook up with, I don't feel like I have to wait for a relationship."

I reminded her of the conversation we had had months earlier with Zoe and Jill. In that discussion, I had asked whether hooking up could lead to a relationship. Absolutely, Jill had said, adding that she had hooked up with a boy a couple of times at parties before the two of them decided to become a couple.

"It works better to hook up first," Jill had argued, "because then you don't have that awkward moment later of 'How do you feel sexually? What do you want to do?' " She and her boyfriend just celebrated their one-year anniversary, she had said, as if that settled the question.

Obviously, this generation isn't the first to treat sex casually. But I remembered thinking at the time that there is casual, and there is casual. Jill had made it seem as if hooking up was on par with shaking hands on a first date. I asked Anna what she thought. Her response told me that she saw hooking up not as an introduction to something more permanent but as a temporary replacement for what she wanted.

"When some people go to sleep at night, they may fantasize about getting it on, but I fantasize about having a relationship," she said. "I wish it was like I hear it used to be. I think, Wouldn't it be nice if this guy I like liked me enough to ask me out? I hope that will happen before the end of high school. Or at least in college.

"Maybe older guys will be more willing to have a relationship."

"[My dad] tries to show me off to other people and I want to say, 'What is there for you to show off? You haven't been here.' But I don't want to mess up what we have. Just being with him makes me happy."
—MIEKA, SIXTEEN

To Mieka and her friends, relating to guys was not so much a contest as a takeover, sometimes hostile, sometimes friendly. Mieka, whose father never lived with her, wanted to make darn sure she could find a boy who would give her what her father rarely had: attention, or at least something resembling attention, and nice things.

Her life, on the surface, did not look much like Sienna's or Anna's.

She was a junior at a public high school in Washington, D.C., with a pre-dominantly African-American student population. The school's tan interior walls badly needed painting, many locker doors wouldn't shut and the big round clocks on the classroom walls rarely showed the right time. By eleventh grade, the year I followed her, many of the boys at school had dropped out or landed in jail, leaving twice as many girls as boys. New teachers who arrived full of enthusiasm frequently left after only a year or two.

Mieka's father had never married her mother and stopped by only occasionally to see his only daughter. She lived with her mother and a step-father to whom she was not particularly close. Her mom and stepdad held steady jobs in the federal government, and most of their salaries went toward paying the mortgage and keeping up their split-level brick house in a quiet D.C. neighborhood of middle-class homes. Unlike Sienna and Anna, Mieka didn't have much money to spend on clothes or movies, and she had never been to a party like the ones those girls described.

But when it came to guys, Mieka's attitude, strategies and language closely resembled those of the better-off white girls. She knew the kind of boy she wanted and wasn't afraid to go after him. She would play him, shrug off any effort on his part to make a commitment and avoid any word, such as "boyfriend," that might hint at deeper feelings.

I met Mieka through a young woman named Camille Harris, who taught sex education at a Boys & Girls Club in a predominantly black, middle-class section of northeast Washington. A recent graduate of Hampton University, in Hampton, Virginia, Harris was a pretty, pixie-like young woman who, I had been told, was very popular with the teenagers who frequented the club. Her workshops about sexuality and sexual health—stressing abstinence as one but not the only option—were ostensibly for fifth- through eighth-graders, but older teens found reasons to "stop by."

As she and I sat on sagging couches in her basement office, waiting for Mieka to arrive and watching with interest the antics of a stray mouse, she tried to describe for me the environment in which girls like Mieka were growing up. "As early as elementary school, they're pretty knowledgeable about the mechanics of sex, though not always," she said. "The story I always tell is about a sixth-grade girl, twelve years old, asking me, 'Miss Camille, if a woman and two men are having a threesome, with one man's penis going into her vagina and the other man's in her . . .'"

"Butt?" Harris had supplied the word.

"Yeah, butt. If that happened, would the penises touch?"

Harris shook her head as if she still couldn't believe what she had heard. "What really got me," she said, "was that none of the other girls in the group were shocked. They just listened. Where in the world have these girls been exposed to a threesome?"

As her young charges moved into high school, Harris said, their interest in the physical, as opposed to emotional, aspects of relating to boys became more pronounced. They would talk about having physical fights with boys, or with other girls over boys. She tried to persuade them to think about what kind of a boy they'd like as a friend, and all they wanted to talk about was a boy as trophy. She had heard similar talk when she was a student at Hampton, she said, where hooking up was "out of control."

"It's this 'Guys can do it, so why can't we?' thing, here and at Hampton. Girls see neediness as a weakness, and it has created this weird thing with relationships."

Minutes later, Mieka arrived, a full-figured sixteen-year-old carefully put together in a canary-yellow sweater, black pants and black heels trimmed in silver, and with perfect braids. Harris had told me that Mieka, vice-president of a young leadership program at the club, was remarkably poised, and I immediately saw that she was right. Mieka introduced me to two classmates from school, Monica and Tonya, both in jeans and

T-shirts, and offered to go out and pick up pizza for all of us while I started interviewing her friends.

"They see more action than I do," she said over her shoulder as she left.

Tonya, a tall, skinny, seventeen-year-old, began by telling me about two recent high school graduates whom she was "talking to," Carter and Robert. She had been to bed with both of them and enjoyed, as Sienna did, keeping boys on a string. Part of her wanted to settle down with one guy but another part of her, again like Sienna, worried how that would play with her friends. "I want to be a committed person," she said, "and I'm thinking about cutting it off with one of them. But what if the other one walks out on me? If you don't have a boyfriend and your friends do, they tell all their stories and you don't have anything to tell."

I turned to Monica, a curvy girl in jeans and a black T-shirt with a sequined front that read "Meow." "Are you in love with anyone?" I asked.

"Who loves people?" she parried. Then she answered my question: She was currently "seeing" Mark and Jerome and, oh yes, a friend of Jerome's and last but certainly not least, a girl named Jill who attended college in southern Virginia. "I've been interested in girls for a while," she said.

Later, in response to another question, she said she goes after girls or guys with the same assertiveness. "My nickname is Cat, and if you don't love me back, I scratch. I'm wild."

When Mieka returned to the club with pizza, it was her turn to confess. She lost her virginity at fourteen, she said, and had four other short relationships over the next two years before meeting Dewayne, a university art student whom she was seeing at the moment.

Keith, an eighteen-year-old neighbor, was her first lover. She was living on and off with her grandmother at the time—had been in fact since fifth grade, when Grandma was put on kidney dialysis and needed someone to help her around the house. Early on the evening of a family funeral, Keith, whom Mieka had known for several years, had stopped by the house. He visited for a while, then pulled her aside and asked if she wanted to ride out to Maryland with him later to visit his apartment. She agreed and shortly after Grandma fell asleep, took her house key, sneaked out and returned in the morning before Grandma got up. That first night, when Keith asked if she wanted to have sex, she said yes. "I did it to see how it would feel," she says. "I didn't think nothing of it before, but after I did it, I felt exposed. I said, 'What did I do? Where did I go wrong?'"

Losing one's virginity, for even the most confident girls, is not like losing one's cell phone or car keys. They can't pick up another "V-card" in a kiosk at the mall. Boys may be eager to shed the label, but girls are not because, for reasons both cultural and biological, it feels like they're closing the door on childhood or, as one girl put it, "like death." Once they do it, they want to put it behind them and find that they can't, at least not immediately.

Mieka's misgivings over what she had done with Keith didn't stop her, however, from continuing to slip out to see him. Sex wasn't the draw. As she recalled, "The first time it was painful, the second time not so much. I guess I got some pleasure out of it, but it didn't make me closer to him." Romance didn't have any hold on her, either. "I don't go in for all that holding hands and stuff," she said.

What kept her wanting him was that he wanted *her* and, unlike her father, regularly showed her that. He would give her money like she imagined other dads gave their daughters, cash that enabled her to purchase the boot-cut jeans and miniature purses that she coveted. He listened to her when she needed to complain to someone about the responsibility she felt for her grandmother. She and Keith could talk easily, she said, without "catching feelings" or getting emotional. Her use of the phrase "catching feelings" surprised me; until that moment, I had heard it used only by white girls to describe what they hoped to avoid by hooking up rather than dating. Mieka was saying the same thing.

Here was the kicker: She broke off the relationship with Keith after a couple of months. He continued to call, but she didn't return his calls. The only reason she could suggest was "I loved him, but wasn't in love with him." As I learned more about her history after Keith, I realized there was more to it. She liked Keith all right, and longed to love him as well as be loved by him. But she was afraid that if she did give him her heart, he would disappoint her, much as her father had. She needed him but suspected she couldn't count on him.

Jonetta Rose Barras wrote about this phenomenon in her book *Whatever Happened to Daddy's Little Girl?* Women whose fathers desert them, physically or emotionally, tend later to go from man to man, seeking to fill a hole that Barras says only gets "larger and deeper." Each time a man rejects them, or doesn't come through for them in some way, they think it's because something is wrong with them. So they search out another man to fill the void, only to be disappointed again.

Barras would recognize Mieka's pattern. After Keith, Mieka said, she felt she had no alternative but to keep having sex. "You know what they say," she told me, " 'Once you pop, the fun don't stop.' " She didn't describe what she did with Keith and the four men after him as "hooking up," but that's what it was. Henry, the first after Keith, was memorable only because she'd watch television while they were having sex and then turn over and read a book or magazine. "I think I was somewhere else on those afternoons," she said. Next was Luis, a Metro bus employee— "in uniform," she sighed—who picked her up from school and took her back to his apartment. He was followed by a barber who regularly gave her lunch money and whose name she couldn't remember, and a "forty-something-year-old man" who approached her one afternoon in his white Escalade while she was strolling down a sidewalk with her cousin. She came away from his apartment several times with a little money in her pocket.

Girls the age Mieka was when she first started having sex typically have sex with men a couple of years older, but most of these men were considerably older. Since she was a minor, any one of them could have been charged with statutory rape. When I told her this, she looked puzzled, as well she might. In the black community, she knew, it was not at all uncommon for young girls to have sex with older men. Indeed, national studies show the same tendency. They also show that black girls have intercourse in slightly larger proportions than white girls (though the gap is narrowing), starting at younger ages. Similar proportions of white and black girls report having one-night stands. (Hispanic girls are less likely to have sex and less likely to have one-night stands, although they start having sex at younger ages than white girls.)

Mieka's behavior was far from what her mother, Linda, would have approved had she known. In her early forties, Linda was a commanding presence: tall and big-boned, with a penchant for brightly colored clothes and forthrightness. Where some mothers, like Beth, wish that their daughters could enjoy the kind of social life they did when they were teenagers, Linda wanted Mieka to do anything but what she had done. She had given birth to her first child, Mieka's sister, at fifteen, never intending to marry the father and keeping the baby only at her mother's insistence. Weekdays she took the baby by bus to a babysitter, caught another bus to a vocational high school and reversed her steps in the evening. She didn't get pregnant again until she was twenty-seven, when she had Mieka, her second and last child. Again, she didn't marry the father, this time because Mieka's dad refused. She supported her daughters at first by working two jobs at a time—frying potatoes at McDonald's and bathing elderly patients as a nursing assistant. Eventually, she went to work for the federal government. She also finished two years of college, a fact that both she and Mieka took great pride in.

Sexuality was not something she was comfortable talking about to her daughter. When Mieka got her first menstrual period at nine, Linda sent her to Linda's mother to learn about her cycles and how to take care of herself. "I remember that day as if it were yesterday," Mieka recalls. "I thought I was dying." Mieka realized then that her mother wasn't comfortable talking about sex, and from that day on, "I never told her anything about what I was doing."

Unlike Sienna's and Anna's mothers, who kept up a running dialogue with their daughters about sex and romance, Linda confined her part of any conversation to little lectures, a couple of which she recalled for me the first time we met at her house. We were sitting in a living room that was comfortably furnished with an oversized stuffed sofa and chairs in tones of beige and burgundy. From the dining room, a dark cherry table and high-back chairs glistened with polish. The most striking thing in both rooms was the clear plastic that covered the furniture. How much easier it is to protect sofas than daughters, I thought.

Shortly after Mieka got her period, Linda said, Linda gave her a little speech. "One of these days you're going to meet a guy who wants to love you, touch you and feel you, and pretty soon he'll drop his drawers," she told her daughter. "Don't let him go any farther. Your education's got to come first. Find a guy who says, 'Let's get our careers in order first.' That's a gentleman." Later talks amounted to the same advice, coupled with instructions on the places Mieka could and could not go. "I want to know where she's been, and I'll call to see if she was where she said she was," Linda told me.

Until tenth grade, Mieka had attended Catholic schools where boys and girls acted politely to each other, at least publicly, lest they draw the wrath of strict principals who handed out suspensions like candy at Halloween. Behavior in her public school was anything but respectful, putting her in the position of abandoning what she knew to be right if she wanted to fit in. The week after our interview at the club, I walked the school hallways with her and watched girls dressed in colors of turquoise, pink and yellow flutter around boys like little birds and then, for no apparent reason, slam them against the lockers. They called this odd sight "joning," and Mieka said she was disgusted by it. "There are like a million girls to ten guys here," she sighed. "Look at the way they act; they just be all over the boys."

As we walked into her art class, a tall boy she knew shook his behind at her and she returned the gesture.

She took a seat next to Monica and Tonya, both dressed that day like rappers, in baggy jeans and black leather jackets. She started copying a paragraph out of a textbook when Tonya interrupted her. It seems that Tonya had chosen Carter over Robert the day before, but Robert, when he heard this, had threatened to come over to her house. Tonya had told him not to do that or she would "cut his throat," but he came anyway, at which point she had pulled a pocketknife out of her waistband and nicked his neck. He knocked the knife out of her hand, she said, and they took the fight outside. He left only when her sister came after him with a baseball bat.

There was something sexy about Robert's swagger, Tonya admitted, adding, "I don't like soft boys I can walk over. I like boys who give me a challenge." I thought back to Sienna describing how nice boys gave girls "the yucks." Women, young and old, have forever been attracted to the bad boys of the world, but since when did flirting mean taking them on in a physical fight?

A REAL RELATIONSHIP, SORT OF

Mieka's current interest, Dewayne (she refused to call him her boyfriend), had graduated from her high school the year before. Eighteen then, and

a serious-looking young man with hair plaits, a faint mustache and gold
wire-rimmed glasses, he seemed classier than the other boys at school,
and she had approached him one afternoon while he was working in the
school library.

During a free period one day at school, she filled me in on their relationship's progression. Dewayne was clearly more than a hookup buddy,
though what he was defied labeling. By the end of the first week after they
met, Mieka recalled, she and Dewayne were talking on the telephone
every night. She told him when to call, when to meet her and how long
he could stay with her. Her mother wouldn't allow her to date, so she had
to think up rendezvous sites well away from her neighborhood; Metro
stops were a favorite. Five months passed before she decided to have sex
with him on a weekday at a house that belonged to one of his friends.
They skipped school and arrived separately; he brought condoms.

He scared her once during their first year together, a couple of weeks
before Valentine's Day. They were arguing in the cafeteria after lunch—
she doesn't remember what it was about—and he pushed her forcefully
into a wall. Then he punched the wall next to her face, putting two holes
in the plaster. She ran upstairs and told the principal, who suspended
Dewayne. Mieka didn't press charges, but she did break up with him for
a month. She insisted, however, that he give her a Valentine's Day gift
while they were broken up, and he did, bringing her a teddy bear and
flowers to school during his suspension.

Despite the suspension, Dewayne graduated on time. That summer,
once he got a job before starting college classes, he bought Mieka a cell
phone and several pairs of shoes. He paid her bills and gave her spending money. She told me on my first visit to her school that the coming
November would be their one-year anniversary, and she already knew
what he was giving her because she had made him tell her: a North
Face jacket, worth about two hundred dollars. "He said he bought it out
of love."

Scientists who study romantic relationships in which couples are having sex say that in three out of four, the partners tell each other "I love you."

Do you love Dewayne? I asked Mieka.

"I do love him," she said. "He's the one."

What is love? I asked her.

"It's about feelings, communication, trust. Someone I can take home to my mother, call my best friend."

This sounded like a traditional boyfriend-girlfriend relationship, but something was missing. Suddenly I realized what it was: It was not *what* she said but *how* she said it. She might as well have been reading from a grocery list. Her voice carried not a hint of emotion, her eyes had no sparkle and her mouth was absent that slight smile some girls give when they're asked to describe someone they've fallen for. The same lack of affect I had observed in Sienna was present in Mieka as well.

I asked Mieka if she and Dewayne had plans for an anniversary dinner.

"No, I'll just go over to his house, get the jacket, go home. I'm not the romantic type. When he gives me this stuff, I'm not, like, 'Oh, you're so wonderful.' I expect that from a guy."

What she didn't expect—or had been taught to be wary of, lest it rope her into a hurtful relationship—was love. This wasn't just because of her father's absence. It also came from the older women in her life who described from their past what they called the "hit it and quit it" guys who promised young girls the moon, had sex with them for a while and then vanished. She decided that if a guy was eventually going to "quit it," she should hold her feelings in reserve and demand, at the very least, a North Face jacket.

A conversation with her aunt that she told me about later that year confirmed my impressions. Her aunt, not her mother, was the person she confided in about personal issues. She recalled that when she told her aunt that she was having sex with Keith, her first sexual partner, her aunt's biggest concern—legitimately—was whether he wore a condom.

What else did your aunt say? I asked.

"She asked me if I would want him to be the father of my child," Mieka recalled. "She asked me if he could support my child, pay for the Pampers."

Did she ask you how you felt about him? I asked. Or how you felt about what you were doing?

"No," said Mieka, "we didn't get into all that." Mieka felt relieved at the time to be able to talk to somebody about Keith. But that somebody, her closest adult confidante, had little to offer in the way of helping her understand her real motivations and feelings—or even the possibilities that come with love.

HER FATHER

Mieka's father, Charles, was certainly not someone to whom she could turn for guidance, although she would have liked to. She first talked about him in detail on a day at school when I offered to save her from cafeteria pizza and take her out for lunch. She immediately thought of a nearby fried-chicken joint where she and her dad went once or twice.

The first thing she wanted to tell me that day had nothing to do with him. She said that on the previous Friday, two girls from her school had jumped a boy who had "dissed" one of the girls. And two different girls had jumped another girl who had been "messin' with" one of their boyfriends.

"All the girls ended up going to the hospital," she said. "This school is crazy."

We returned to the subject of her father while waiting for wings and fries.

Her most vivid memories of him were when she was younger and he'd pick her up after school and take her to his girlfriend's house to spend the night. Sometimes they would drop by a certain liquor store on the way and he would show her off to his buddies who hung around the store. He'd ask his pals to go into the store and pick up some candy, juice, ice cream or popcorn, "really anything I wanted." Such goodies might not spell "father" to a girl whose father helped her with homework or coached her soccer team. But they were virtually all that Mieka got from her dad—she mentioned those trips to the liquor store several times over the course of our year—and thus took on a significance far out of proportion to their actual worth. When I realized this, I understood why she associated love from her hookup partners with the cash and gifts they gave her.

As Mieka got older, her dad visited less frequently. Right after she started high school, she learned for the first time, from Linda, her mother, that when Linda gave birth to her and pressed Charles for child support, he balked, forcing the court to order a blood test. Even after the blood test proved his paternity, his support payments were erratic. Mieka told me that day at lunch that he still owed $13,000.

"I guess the thing that bothers me most is he tried to disown me," she said.

People told Mieka that she resembled her father more than her mother, and she was not sure how to take that. "He tries to show me off to other people and I want to say, 'What is there for you to show off? You haven't been here.' But I don't want to mess up what we have. Just being with him makes me happy."

As we walked through an alley back toward school, Mieka volunteered, "I guess the older boyfriends fill some spots somewhere." And what would those spots be? Something besides trinkets and clothes? "They spend time with me, talk to me."

I joined two of her teachers who were eating lunch in an empty classroom. One of them, her entrepreneurship instructor, had taught in the school for forty years; the other, an English teacher, for fifteen.

"Something has made our kids become very needy," the English teacher said. "They're looking for something to fill that neediness. They want a companion, but no one ever talks to them about what true companionship is. They think it's all about sex."

Her colleague nodded. "Or they think they're in love because of what the guys buy them. A lot of them have been taught only that men are supposed to provide, that that's what men are good for."

For Christmas, Dewayne gave Mieka a pair of New Balance boots, and this time she gave him something also: two pairs of expensive jeans and Calvin Klein cologne, purchased with money she begged from her mother. On her birthday three weeks later, he gave her half of a gold heart on a chain. He wore the other half. The transaction took place at a subway stop in Washington and lasted all of twenty minutes because she was on her way to the Boys & Girls Club. The club was the one place she could discuss her life with adults who listened and seemed to understand, and it was telling that she wanted to be there rather than with Dewayne. "I be too busy to really be together with him. He understands."

Or perhaps he didn't. Near the end of the school year, he called off their relationship, saying he was interested in a classmate at art school. For a couple of weeks "I felt, like, empty," Mieka recalled.

But then he telephoned and said his new honey wasn't ready for a committed relationship. He wanted Mieka back. I was surprised that after he hurt her she'd agree to go back. But he filled a part of the hole left by her father; without him it would have been completely empty.

"I said I wasn't going to be his run-back girl," she said. "But we're seeing each other again. His mom gave him a car. He'll pick me up and we'll go to his house. I'm trying as hard as I can to make it last."

She had invested a lot more time with Dewayne than with the other men she had known, and although she wouldn't admit it, more emotion. She had invited him over to her house once, around Christmastime, to meet her mom, who liked him (while at the same time warning her not to get "too serious"). She had visited his mother at their home several times and liked her, even though, in Mieka's view, she tried to control her son too much. Dewayne could be petty and argumentative, even violent, and because he had had an abusive father, Mieka worried about the latter. But he had proven also to be honest and generous.

Another plus: He satisfied her in bed. "The sex was nothing to brag about at first," she said, "but it got better. Now it's pleasurable all the time." This was no small thing. In fact, she admitted, "If we didn't have sex, we wouldn't have so many feelings for each other and I probably wouldn't be with him."

Our last day together came shortly after school got out for the summer. We sat in her living room on the plastic-covered sofa. She brought me up to date on her two friends. Tonya had gotten pregnant by the guy she stabbed, and had had an abortion. Monica had broken up with several boys and was now seeing her girlfriend more regularly. Mieka looked at what her friends were doing—just as Jamie, Sienna and, to a certain extent, Anna did—and declared herself satisfied with Dewayne, for the moment.

"We are together, but we don't go together," she said. "At least we don't say that we do. If we said it, it would seem like we were married."

College

"I wanted to prove I still had the upper hand."
—NICOLE, NINETEEN

N icole took revenge on James, a former hookup partner, in two quick strokes, one week apart, during the fall of her sophomore year at George Washington University, in Washington, D.C.

She and James, a prep school graduate from Boston, had hung out together for about a month early in their freshman year. To an outsider it would have appeared they were enjoying a relationship, but they called it an exclusive hookup, meaning they didn't hook up with anyone else but remained uncommitted emotionally. Allegedly.

After winter break freshman year, James had stopped returning Nicole's calls. A strikingly pretty girl with dark-brown eyes and straight, reddish-brown hair, Nicole had no trouble resuming an active social life. But she didn't forget James or his treatment of her.

The next year, late on a Saturday night in September, just hours after I had left her at a party, she ended up at his friend's house with her girlfriends, somewhat drunk. A small group assembled to go out for pancakes, James and Nicole among them. She started flirting with him on the

way over and ended up, after pancakes, having sex with him back in his
fraternity house. The next morning he begged her to stay longer. She
didn't. As she walked out the door she smiled. Yes, I did it, she said to
herself. I got him.

She found out how much she had gotten to him the next weekend. At
two o'clock Saturday morning, as she headed for her sorority house after
a night of bar-hopping, she got a "U busy?" call—in plain English, a
solicitation—on her cell phone. It was James. "Why don't we meet up?"
he asked. She changed direction, walked to his fraternity house. They had
sex again and fell asleep.

Several hours later, as she prepared to leave, he asked her, "What do
we do about this?"

She stuffed her clothes into a big purse, pulled on some blue flannel
sleep pants he offered and a North Face jacket.

"We do nothing," she said. "I got what I wanted." Then she walked
back to her sorority house.

A few days later, she tossed his pants in the trash.

The sex wasn't great, Nicole admitted later, but that's not why she had
spent the night either time. "I wanted to prove I still had the upper hand.
I knew he could get a lot of girls, and I was playing his own game. I felt
nothing for him the whole time. I just turned my mind off."

Having the upper hand, making the better deal, outfoxing your
opponent—the campaign to capture the young man of one's choice and
then drop him at will assumes a decidedly more serious tone once high
school girls get to college. Using sex—intercourse, especially—to get revenge makes a young woman feel powerful. With guys, there's always
the risk of feeling powerless, and she can't afford that: She needs to be
powerful in order to both attract guys and keep them at arm's length so
she can stay focused on herself and her studies.

To older eyes, college hookups, drunken parties, the bar scene and
even the bizarre event known as the date auction may appear merely to

be different shapes of a last hurrah before jobs, mortgages and the other perils of adulthood. Cosseted and controlled by parents in their earlier years, students, female and male, are on their own for the first time, living on campuses where there are no obvious rule makers and few rules except those they impose on themselves. They can hardly be blamed for wanting to sample everything in sight. As Patty, Nicole's best friend, put it, "Our favorite nights are those with lots of giggling, when you can say anything to anybody because you're drunk, dance on the tables or pee outside on the pavement. What's the point of college if you don't do this? We'll never get to do this again. If I'm thirty and still doing this, lock me up and take my kid away."

But it's not just fun and games they're looking for, girls say privately. It's fun and games with someone of their choosing. And that's serious business.

Positioned in the middle of *U.S. News & World Report*'s one hundred top-ranked universities, GW does not enjoy the academic reputation of Duke, which consistently stays near the top of the list. GW's eighteen Division I sports teams also cannot compete with Duke's overall athletic success. But GW has something Duke does not, something that attracts a particular kind of student, and that is a connection to politics and power that is unchallenged. Within walking distance of the White House and the President's executive office buildings, it owns sixty-six acres of land in D.C., making it the second largest landowner in the city after the federal government. Its adjunct faculty members are drawn from the highest levels of government and the media. GW's graduate programs in political science and public affairs are among the most selective in the country, and its list of notable alumni is impressive, from J. Edgar Hoover to former Secretary of State Colin Powell.

This access to, and interest in, political power, combined with GW's well-known medical school and presence in the heart of an urban area, attracts students who are engaged in the world and eager to make their mark on it—if not in politics then in other high-profile fields. These students, like their counterparts at Duke, tend to come from families of means: With tuition, room and board at about $45,000 a year, GW is one of the priciest universities in the country. So what you find among GW's 10,000 undergraduates are many who have been given much and expect to give back much to the world. Nicole was one of them.

I met Nicole, nineteen at the time, over dinner at an Italian restaurant on the GW campus at the beginning of her sophomore year. Before arriving at school, she had lived all her life in a gracious, split-level house in an established Dallas community of similar homes on a flat, wide, tree-lined street. She and her older sister, Cleo, attended top private schools; after high school, she had followed Cleo to GW, wooed by a full academic scholarship.

The neighborhood in which she grew up was unnaturally quiet, but it was a different story inside her house. Her parents, Daphne, of Greek heritage, and Niko, a Greek native, were generous to the core—generous with their friends and with their opinions. Nicole learned early that she had to scream to be heard.

In an upstairs hallway of her home, hung side by side, is a sequence of five framed photographs of Nicole as a toddler, standing in her crib, her face in a state of uncontrolled rage. Nicole, her mother says, was "hell on wheels."

"If I had had her first, I would not have had a second child," Daphne said, chuckling during an interview. "She didn't sleep through the night until she was three. She'd sit in the dark, rocking away in her crib, yelling and screaming."

Nicole was one of those children who, early on, assumed that people would love her. A certain family story is told and retold: One day when Nicole and her sister were in preschool, Niko, a financial analyst who worked at home, arrived to pick them up. Both girls were standing in line with other girls, waiting their turn to get a drink from the water fountain. As Cleo approached the front of the line, two six-year-olds moved in front of her, and Cleo said nothing. When it was Nicole's turn at the fountain, two other girls tried to do the same thing to her. Nicole placed her four-year-old hands on her hips and blocked them. "I'm here next," she said loudly, "and you're not getting anything before I do."

In her all-girl high school, a school where two of every three students made perfect scores on their Advanced Placement tests and virtually all graduates go to college, Nicole was a fierce competitor. In matters of the heart, she was the same: At summer camp after ninth grade, she set her sights on William, the best-looking camp counselor, and quickly won him over. He was the first and only guy she called a boyfriend until midway through her sophomore year at GW.

William, also from Dallas and three years ahead of her in school, went off to the University of Texas at the end of that summer, but she continued to date him when he came home over the next three years and when, with her mother's knowledge, she sneaked over to UT. After he started dating someone else at college, she didn't bow out of the picture but simply assumed he'd eventually come back to her. Their love, she recalled, was both frail and fierce.

"We couldn't keep from holding hands and touching each other. We'd be out with other people but only talk to each other. No one could crack our world."

She knew what she would and wouldn't do sexually. She would make out with William, doing everything but intercourse. "I wasn't ready for that," she said. Her best friend, Libby, had sex with a longtime boyfriend the year Nicole and Libby were high school seniors. Nicole called her mother, crying, when she found out. "They're not good for each other," Nicole said. "She's making too many mistakes for him."

With the end of high school approaching, Nicole considered and then rejected the idea of enrolling at UT to be near William. He had said once that he wanted a wife who would stay home to raise the children.

That wasn't for her; she had plans to become a doctor. In addition, she couldn't see herself doing what Libby had done and following a boyfriend to college. She thought that would be like "handing my life over to him."

Shortly before final exams, William, who had wanted her to join him, warned her, "We'll never be done." On the day of her senior exams, she cried on and off for fourteen hours.

Three months later she was enrolling in biology and Spanish classes at GW and, on weekends, "getting out there and getting known."

For some girls that would have presented a challenge, given the presence of 10,000 other undergraduates. But Nicole had allies because she joined a sorority. Daphne had been surprised when her willful freshman daughter joined what was, in essence, one big clique that valued conformity. Nicole saw pledging as a no-brainer. In her mind, a sorority wasn't that different from a girls' school and had two distinct advantages: lots of occasions where she could wear pretty dresses, and a steady parade of fraternity boys to choose from. She sounded a bit defensive when I mentioned her mother's reaction to her decision. "Sorority life is not who I am," she said. "It's a childish game. I don't take it seriously."

Sorority life may not have determined who she was directly, but it did help determine the company she kept. Many of the boys she hooked up with belonged to fraternities, and fraternities hosted many of the parties at GW, as they do on other campuses—occasions given names like Pimps and Prostitutes, and Playboy Bro's and Ho's (required dress for guys being silk robes, for girls, bunny suits). Fraternities also provided booze and, if partying at a private club, bouncers who looked the other way when underage sisters showed up.

Kappa Sigma provided James at a Halloween party.

Nicole was dressed as a Red Sox baseball player and he, it turned out, loved the Sox.

"Hello, who are you?" he asked.

She had seen him around campus but hadn't taken the time to look him up on Facebook, an online community of college students from several hundred colleges and universities. "Oh, the mystery guy," she cooed.

They hung out a lot over the next month, eating lunch together, talking baseball, even getting their flu shots together. She wasn't in love with him but, much like Jamie with Jake, relished the fact that people would meet her and say, "Oh, you're the girl James is with." The closest she ever came to sounding sentimental about him, as she recounted this time to me a year later, was when she said he was "comfort."

"Like a stuffed bear, perhaps?" I joked.

"Yeah, something like that. We'd do things together but we were never together." Without the conventions of dating that she had enjoyed with William, she really didn't know how to explain what she had with James.

One Saturday night at a Washington club, Nicole, somewhat tipsy, brought up a subject with James that had weighed on her mind for a while.

"Have you ever had sex?" she asked.

"Yeah," James said. "Seven times. And you?"

Nicole had not but was ready to. At eighteen, she was older by a year than the age at which girls, on average, first have sex. She didn't know that, but she did know that she was embarrassed to admit that she was a college freshman and still a virgin. Virginity in college implied that, no matter how hot you were, you didn't want or like sex. "I was tired of waiting," she said. "James and I were together, and I wanted to know what it was like."

She told me that on that night, she and James had taken a Yellow Cab from the club back to his dorm, and that she was wearing a black camisole, blue jeans and a bright red tweed jacket with tiny zippers on each sleeve that her sister had purchased for her in Paris. She described

James's room, his bed and the condoms he kept in the drawer of his bedside table. I was surprised by how much she remembered but read later
that women always remember in great detail the first time they had sex,
even women who take so many men to bed that they forget the other
names and faces. I suspect that it's not just lost maidenhood that etches
that one time in their minds, but also the first-time union of the physical and the emotional—a powerful reaction that young women often
aren't expecting.

After James and Nicole had sex that first time, he asked her, "Are you
okay?" She said she was. The next morning she walked back to her dorm
alone, in the previous night's clothes. Although the sex had been nothing special, she had a smile on her face as she did "the stride of pride,"
a phrase some girls use to replace the old "walk of shame."

Her telling of this story reminded me of Jamie at Duke early in her
freshman year, slipping out of Jake's room on Saturday and Sunday
mornings to return unaccompanied to East Campus. Why did young
women always seem to be the ones making the trip home, without an es-
cort? Did that give them a sense of being more in control—or less?
Nicole said more. "That way, we can leave when we want to." Left un-
said was the fact that it also relieved their partners of showing that they
cared for the girls' well-being.

In the next couple of weeks that year, Nicole and James had sex several times, "trying to get the hang of it," she recalled. Nicole insisted that
he wear a condom every time and that he put it on. She wanted to have
nothing to do with that.

Nicole's account about her early time with James seemed to me at
first to be an example of pure, if unsatisfied, lust. The feeling of lust, a
craving like no other, is separate from love, according to anthropologist
Helen Fisher. Originating in a different part of the brain than romantic
passion, lust motivated our ancestors "to seek sexual union with almost
any semi-appropriate partner," Fisher writes in her book *Why We Love*.

It can be triggered by love but may also spring up on its own and last for a while, apart from any deeper feelings. This is as true for young women as for young men, according to Fisher, although it may not occur as frequently for females.

But as I thought more carefully about how Nicole talked about James, I realized she didn't feel much lust or love for him. Sex with him "felt like something," she told me, "but it wasn't very interactive." She was not the first girl to talk to me about sex in disappointed terms, and that made me sad. Here these girls were, targeting boys, planning and executing their strategies, risking pregnancy, disease and heartbreak—and being let down time and again by sex that wasn't as satisfying as they had hoped it would be. One of their goals, as well as one of their best weapons, wasn't what they expected.

Over winter break that freshman year, James called Nicole at home in Dallas only once, and when they returned to campus, "things just kinda fizzled." She'd run into him and he'd say he was going to phone, but he never did. She wasn't one to sit around and wait, so she plunged back into the hookup scene. And the next year, got him back.

One evening I asked Nicole how many boys she had hooked up with that first year. She looked at Patty, also a sophomore, and started naming names:

"Let's see, there was Rick."

"Then Mark," Patty chimed in.

Nicole continued, "Then Phil and all the SAEs."

The SAEs?

"That's short for the fraternity Sigma Alpha Epsilon."

"Or," said Patty, "Sexual Assault Expected." She grinned.

The recitation continued with Stan the Man, Bob, Randy, Jack, Jasper, Jeremy, Nate and two guys she called Polo Player and Tennis Boy because she couldn't remember their names.

Nicole paused. "There's more, I know there's more. A bunch of us in the sorority counted up. I had the highest number, maybe fifteen or twenty." She also took pride in the fact that she was managing to keep close to an A average in a heavy course load that included economics and several pre-med courses.

She wanted me to know that she might hook up one time or a couple of times with the same guy over a semester, in clubs, cabs or bedrooms, and that hooking up consisted of kissing, petting and, occasionally, oral sex. Her favorite activity was kissing. The peck, the lip-lock, the French kiss, the vacuum kiss ("sucking the air out of your partner"), she had mastered them all. Sometimes, she kissed deeply, with feeling. At other times she just went through the motions: "the hookup kiss," she called it.

In the confusion of the unhooked culture, kissing may signal nothing more than friendship. Or it may resemble the first shot over the bow in a campaign to seduce. Tony, the self-described "player" in the class I taught at GW, and a formidable opponent for any young woman, wrote to me about his experience one night at Lulu's, a bar near campus:

As the person who throws the parties, I found myself kissing several people who came "just to see me." An awkward situation, yet with liquor involved, a tongue kissed seemed minute in the big scheme of things, and the girls would be satisfied.

Then there were the girls who are friends or good acquaintances who decided to let me know they liked me. . . . They would feel stupid and rejected and probably act awkward the next day if I pushed them aside. . . . But with a kiss, it could be chalked up to a funny incident at the club that happened when all of us were drunk.

Then there was the randomness. Two girls who I was dancing with made their tongues ready for my mouth. While these were more sneak attacks than anything, and while I did find them to be really attractive girls, I wasn't all for kissing them. But I did it and then

walked away. I probably kissed ten people. I kissed no one whom I
was interested in. And I didn't go home alone.

LIQUID COURAGE: FUEL FOR THE FIGHT

On a Friday night in January, Nicole and several girlfriends met at the
GW student center to introduce me to the date auction, a charitable fund-
raising event popular with student organizations on campuses around the
country.

The auctions vary in nature—some are sedate and some, like GW's,
anything but. This one, in its third year, featured barely clad freshman
athletes dancing like dogs in heat on an elevated runway as upperclass
students bid on them for a dinner out. Girls bid on guys, guys bid on girls,
and judging by the swaying bodies and slurred speech, almost everyone
was smashed. Nicole and her posse had plans to go to a bar later, so Patty
and a couple of other girls took off for a restroom to finish off a six-pack
first, following unspoken rules of the culture: Girls get drunk with girls,
guys with guys, and the sexes then come together to drink more, flirt,
dance and hook up.

Midway through the auction, Nicole and friends departed for a favorite saloon known as Exchange. With a quick flash of their fake IDs
(Nicole's belonged to her older sister), they squeezed their way into
their generation's prime hunting ground: the bar. Frequently, college-
town bars hire students to promote weekend parties by stuffing mailboxes
and e-mailing classmates. Whether that had been the case on this night
was unclear, but for whatever reason, Exchange was packed.

Nicole knew where to stand to catch a bartender's eye. Normally she
might have waited for a guy to buy her a drink, but on this night she
snagged two gin-and-tonics and maneuvered her way through the crowd
with the confidence of someone who had done this before. Patty followed her into an adjoining room, which was only slightly less crowded,

carrying glasses and a pitcher of draft beer (the saloon boasts thirteen different varieties). If you were going to drink a beer, she told me, you bought a pitcher to share with whoever happened to ask. That way, those under twenty-one, as she was, who were, unlike her, scared to approach the bar, wouldn't miss out on the fun.

The two girls stationed themselves at a small table where a middle-aged waiter in a short-sleeved red shirt was piling empty glasses onto a tray. He managed to stack up a couple of dozen before heading for the kitchen, dodging young drunks.

Nicole pulled her cell phone out and dialed a friend in Dallas to talk about an upcoming visit. How she could hear above the din of the crowd, I'll never know. Patty was on a quest. A couple of nights earlier, at a different bar, she had met a freshman who told her, "The first time I saw you, I knew I wanted to hang out with you." It was not exactly the cleverest pickup line she'd ever heard, but he *was* cute. They had shared a few drinks, and the next thing she knew, it was midmorning the next day and she was lying in her bed clad only in jeans, belt and pearls. The boy's chocolate-brown overcoat was lying on a chair, its owner nowhere to be seen. "Hey, how did I get home?" she had asked her roommate, Ann. Ann didn't have any idea.

Patty hoped on this night to meet the coat's owner. She felt hot, sexy and ready to pick up where they had left off. But she also was afraid of being turned down, thus the beer. "Liquid courage," she and her classmates called it.

Of the hundreds of young women I interviewed about hookup experiences, less than a half-dozen said they were sober at the time. Some drank for the exhilarating high, others because everyone around them was drinking, others to relax and still others, like Patty, to quiet the cautionary voices in their heads. Surveys consistently show that girls experience more negative feelings in sexual situations than guys do. But a pitcher of beer can do wonders to ease fear and feelings of insecurity.

Plus, as Patty explained to me, if you wake up the next day alongside someone who is "coyote ugly" ("You'd rather gnaw off your arm than be with him"), you can slough it off by saying, "I was sooooo wasted. I don't remember anything."

A hangover is a small price to pay for exoneration.

Alcohol is the social lubricant that fuels the unhooked culture, beginning in high school and particularly in college, where intercourse becomes more common. Moderate drinking among college-aged students has declined slightly over the last two decades, but binge drinking, defined as five or more drinks in a row for men, four or more for women, has remained constant. In a Harvard School of Public Health study of 119 four-year colleges, half of the students said they drank to get drunk, and nearly half said they had had four or five drinks in one sitting within the previous two weeks. This can't be chalked up to ignorance: Students have heard about the dangers of drinking since fourth-grade D.A.R.E. classes, just as they've learned, since sixth grade, the possible physical consequences of unprotected sex. Many of them seem unable to moderate either drinking or sex—which, of course, feed on each other.

Binge drinking starts in earnest in college. One rarely wanders through a dorm or frat house late on a Thursday or Friday evening without coming across drinking games such as "Beer Pong" or "Never Have I Ever." The latter is a favorite with girls who sit in a circle, beverages nearby. The first girl lifts her drink for a toast and says something like, "Never have I ever had sex in the ocean," or "Never have I ever hooked up with Billy." Anyone in the circle who has in fact done what the other girl says she hasn't done, has to take a swig. As many as four out of five college students take part in at least one drinking game in college, according to studies.

Young women who play such games drink, on average, five drinks per game, according to one study at a midsized midwestern university. In fact, young women's overall alcohol consumption has risen over the past ten years to where it almost matches that of young men. Every spring, a handful of college newspapers can be counted on to carry stories about sorority formals being shut down early by those who manage the art museums, plush hotels or other venues where the formals are held because a few girls passed out or vomited in public.

Yet when you talk to girls about drinking, they often say they don't have a problem. (Sienna was an exception.) In one national study, nine of every ten women who reported what amounted to binge drinking nevertheless labeled themselves light to moderate drinkers.

During my first few visits to nightclubs, I noticed girls and boys taking digital photos of each other with their cell phones as the time for "last call" at the bar approached. Puzzled, I asked a medical student about it one evening in a Durham bar. Throwing back his fourth shot, he explained, "We need the pictures so we can remember who we were with the night before." The technology makes it a snap: They record the person's phone number in their phone, snap a photo and add whatever text they want ("Saturday night at Exchange"). The next day they can pull up the previous night in an instant. And if someone they don't know calls them, a glance at the accompanying photo will remind them of who the caller is.

Several explanations have been suggested for excessive drinking: intoxication observed at home; the cultural assumption that drinking is a rite of passage; drink specials and other promotions at clubs and bars near campus; lax enforcement of the legal drinking age. Health advocates point a finger at alcohol manufacturers who target young women by advertising the fruity taste of so-called girlie drinks. They also note that parents and other influential adults are not as likely to get upset at alcohol as cigarettes or illegal drugs because, chances are, those adults drink, too.

But blaming hookups on alcohol misses a larger point: Booze doesn't cause college students to jump into bed with each other, it simply makes it easier for them to do something they think they want to do, knowing it is not necessarily good for them. Young women would like to win over young men without losing their hearts or their self-esteem, and hooking up is one way to do that. However, no matter how often they've hooked up, the prospect makes some of them uncomfortable and a bit scared. Pretty soon, they're relying on booze to approach the dance floor, a partner and a bed. It's a vicious cycle: They drink to have sex but get little pleasure from the sex so the next time they drink again, hoping the sex will be better.

The more they drink, the more likely they are to have unprotected sex, fall dangerously ill, be involved in an automobile accident or be sexually assaulted. Sexual assault is considered by some researchers young women's biggest risk because when they're drunk, they may be unable to communicate effectively what they want or don't want to do. According to Leslie Campis, a psychology professor and sexual assault counselor at Emory University, the young woman who binge drinks increases her risk by at least fifty percent of being sexually assaulted. In a Harvard study of campus rapes, three out of four women were judged to have been too drunk to give consent or resist.

The GW date auction provided an example of what Campis and other experts have written about. This was the auction where Morgan and other freshman water polo players sold themselves to a guy who paid a hundred dollars to take the young women out to dinner at a later date. Morgan, completely stoned on a combination of liquor and Xanax, ended up that night in the bed of a man she barely knew, who had sex with her while she was passed out. She blamed the incident on alcohol. Over that cup of coffee on campus four months later, she tried to remember the specifics of the night.

"Like, I had been talking to this guy and we were just, like, friends or whatever, but, like, I don't really remember what happened, and then I just blacked out. I remember getting back to my room. . . . I ended up sleeping with him."

Did she feel violated? I asked. The law in the District of Columbia, as in many jurisdictions, states that if a person is too drunk to give consent to intercourse, she or he has been sexually assaulted.

"That's the thing I, like, kind of debate once I look back at it," she said. "It's hard, because he's, like, a pretty respectable guy. And, like, he was completely sober. . . . He obviously knew I was drunk, but I don't think he knew I was drunk to the point where I was blacked out. . . . That night a lot of my girlfriends on the water polo team did end up, like, being with guys.

"Everyone there was, like, completely wasted. . . . There's a difference between high school and college. It's definitely a step up alcohol-wise, because, at least from my perspective, I never drank in high school. Like, I drank in high school, but not nearly as much as you're kind of forced to by the culture of college, you know? I've definitely become, like, a drinker in college. I'm pretty much a champ at it."

Morgan was convinced that Greek life had a lot to do with how much she drank.

"Last year, the Delta house had a party," she said, "and we were walking around with beer up to our ankles. Drinking has definitely become part of my life. And it's caused me to do stupid shit. . . ."

Morgan hadn't been able to bring herself to admit her misgivings to any of her friends because they all seemed to be having such a good time when they drank. So she had turned to her mother, who had contacted a psychiatrist at GW's hospital. All he did when she visited his office, Morgan said, was prescribe medication. Her situation was far from unique, according to campus health officials; with college mental-health services often underfinanced and understaffed, many students suffer silently, drop out or return home.

Party life on campus doesn't affect all girls equally. Someone as strong-willed as Nicole knew her limits and usually honored them. For whatever reason, Morgan was unable to either set limits or hold to them.

By midnight at Exchange, Patty had had plenty to drink. Brown Coat Boy had been found and had brushed her off, so she flirted with a tall, curly-haired blond wearing a dark baseball cap, who marched her in the direction of a corner couch. She returned to me later and launched into a whispered, drunk narrative of her life in high school as the girlfriend of a popular lacrosse player. "I used to be confident, but I'm not any more," she said. "My boyfriend, at Georgetown University, told me this summer we needed to cool things off. I thought all this partying and hooking up would make me feel better and sometimes it does, but it makes me wonder whether I'll ever have a real relationship." As she started to elaborate, Curly Blond approached and motioned toward the couch. She rolled her eyes at me and took his hand.

When I lingered in clubs such as Exchange, students I didn't know invariably approached me, wanting to know what I was doing there. When they found out, they usually had a story to tell. This night was no different. After Patty left, a gorgeous young woman with long, flowing red hair and hoop earrings told me she had just come from "a real date" with a guy who had cooked dinner.

"He grilled steak," she said. "I have no interest in him, but hey, it was steak."

She said she had been hooking up all fall with another guy and although "he isn't too bright, I'm starting to feel emotionally attached to him." This worried her, but not too much, as she had plans to go abroad soon and that would conveniently put an end to things. As soon as she left, a short guy with straight brown hair that kept falling in his face came up and began talking about a girl he had hooked up with whom he was crazy about. Problem was, she wasn't crazy about him. "I cry a lot about this," he said, and he looked as if he might burst into tears on the spot. I was grateful when a buddy of his walked over and gently pulled him away.

I was moved not only by such stories but by the desire of the story-tellers to share them with a stranger—an indication that they were look-ing for some direction in how to think about circumstances that were confusing, even intimidating.

Shortly before I left Exchange that winter night, the owner ap-proached me to chat and, I suspect, make sure I wasn't there to bust him for serving alcohol to minors. His bouncers check IDs, he said, but, and he waved his hand around the room, "You and I both know that kids will drink. As long as they're all GW students, and they're here, they'll be safe." He motioned toward Nicole and her friends. "Aren't they great?" he said. "I've got three daughters, eight, eleven and twelve. I hope they all go to GW, just like these girls."

I took my leave, walking across a floor sticky with liquor and pass-ing the red-shirted waiter now on his umpteenth trip to the kitchen with empty glasses. I waved down a cab, and as I was sliding onto the back-seat, two very drunk blondes piled in next to me without asking. The cab-driver asked the girls where they were headed. "Twenty-first and H," said Girl Number One. "Twenty-third and H," said Number Two.

They didn't speak to each other or to me. The cabbie stopped on Twenty-first, and Number One girl opened the right rear door and lit-erally fell onto the pavement. As she picked herself up and staggered to-ward a tall brick building, she yelled that the friend she left behind would pay for her ride. The cabbie proceeded two blocks, and as he pulled up to the curb, Number Two girl flew out the cab, running toward her dorm without paying.

"Girls do this a lot." The cabbie sighed.

"Then why do you pick them up?" I asked.

"I just want them to get home safely," he said.

When he dropped me off at home, I gave him enough cash to cover our three fares, pondering the fact that to ordinary working stiffs, these girls were the cream of the crop.

CHICKS BEFORE DICKS

For Nicole, the night at Exchange was uneventful. Not so a party a few weeks before, where she ran into James and one of his frat brothers, the exotic-looking, brown-skinned Nate.

Except for her trysts with James in the fall, sophomore year had been relatively tame. In danger of failing physics during the first semester a potential disaster for a pre-med student—she had resolved to spend more time on her studies. But she couldn't see not enjoying any action at all and so had been hooking up on and off with Nate.

At the party, she and Nate kissed for a while, then circulated separately. Nicole wasn't surprised when James then approached her, but she was taken aback by what he said.

"Miss Nicole," he announced loudly, "I despise you."

Pretty wasted by this point and ready to take him on, she followed him to the bar, yelling at him until Patty appeared and steered her away.

Despite her reconquest of James a couple of months before, Nicole hadn't been able to get him out of her head. She would see him on campus flirting with girls and instinctively want to punch him or them. She knew she had gotten even with him this year, she told me one night at a restaurant, but that didn't completely erase her feeling of having been used or her disappointment at having lost her virginity to him.

"I still know I was number eight," she said.

"And that," said Patty, who was with us, "is what sucks."

While some young women can sleep with men and not become attached, many cannot. Scientists who study the endocrine system suggest one reason for that. When female mammals engage in intercourse, the hormone oxytocin is released in large amounts. Oxytocin, usually associated with the release of breast milk during childbirth, stimulates a caring instinct during or after intercourse, apparently more in women than in men. Though the research is still new, there's a good chance that, as one scientist put it, "you're specific to a man as soon as you have sex." Severing that bond can be emotionally very difficult, as Nicole was finding out.

An hour after their shouting match, Nicole saw James dancing and making out with Patty's roommate, Ann, and when James and Ann disappeared from the party, Nicole's mind spun. Had Ann gone home with him? Ann was her friend; even in the unhooked culture, friends didn't do that to each other, at least not in the open. Again, Nicole's fighting instincts surfaced, and again, Patty talked her down, telling her how foolish she was being.

"Nicole," she said, "turn off the stupid box."

"I needed her to say that," Nicole admitted later in telling this story.

The next day, after their public argument, James posted an "away" message on his computer that anyone could read, saying, "I hate drama and everyone who perpetuates it."

Nicole shot back a quick e-mail: "Fuck off. You made out with Ann on the dance floor." A few other angry e-mails were exchanged until Nicole, with continual help from Patty, calmed down.

As dates and serious boyfriends have dwindled in number, girls have become each other's life-support systems. One college newspaper columnist put it this way: "The long-term relationship has been replaced by the long-term friendship." Without their parents or other authorities around telling them what they can and cannot do, college women depend on their gal pals to push them out there and then protect them from going too far. They've even coined a phrase capturing their sisterhood: "Chicks before dicks," an in-your-face response to the fraternity-inspired motto "Bro's before ho's."

"My girlfriends in college are my life," Patty told me. Cleo, Nicole's sister, confessed that when her roommate and best friend considered dropping out of GW and returning home and then decided to stay, "that was lots more important than my boyfriend telling me he loved me for the first time."

Occasionally I wondered if these girls ever took time out to be by themselves and reflect, apart from their girlfriends. They swarmed in clusters on the quad, in the coffee shop and in the dorm—piling in threes and fours onto a single bed and laughing at all the crazy stuff they had done that day. They sent instant messages to each other on the computer (a kind of giant conference call) and text-messaged each other on their cell phones a dozen times a day. They'd go to the Web domain Facebook and write on each other's "virtual wall" things like, "Nicole love, the hot boys have had you long enough, I want you back here with me," and "Hope studying is going well bc my calc class is kicking my ass." They'd add each other's names and photos to their Facebook pages; typically their buddy lists would hold several hundred names. The photos they put up of themselves on the pages were telling: In Nicole's, she was grinning into the camera as Patty kissed her, the top of a liquor bottle between them.

The passion that college girls expressed for their *amies*, and the disdain they showed toward guys, reminded me of the documented feelings of middle-class young women in the late nineteenth century, who lived within a far more gender-rigid society. Today's women have male buddies, at least many of them do, but feel a deep need nonetheless for female copilots to help them navigate their ill-defined social terrain.

Watching a team of young women prepare to take over a bar was like watching a military campaign. Hours before the assault, they would figure out where the boys they most wanted to see would be. They'd discuss uniform, gear and strategy. Each girl always took a battle buddy, as Nicole did with Patty, to scout out guys, gather intelligence, report back and, most important, protect her from shooting at the wrong target or taking fire. It was a bit like the Air Force, when pilots station a copilot right behind them to "watch their six," or their back. In the unhooked culture of a coed school, they needed someone to "watch their six," and girls like Morgan, who didn't have that someone, could get into big trouble.

Shelley Taylor, a psychologist at the University of California–Los Angeles, has done research that helps explain this bonding. In certain stressful situations, she writes—and the unhooked culture is nothing if not stressful—the female response is less the male's "fight or flight" than "tend and befriend." Animal data, including human data, strongly suggest that anxious females cope by seeking support from other females, a tendency thought to be based in the primitive need to protect offspring.

Sometimes, girls will pull their pals right into the culture with them. This was an example:

A blonde and a brunette entered the bathroom at the nightclub Lulu's one Friday night. Brunette dashed into a stall; Blonde evaluated herself in the mirror.

"So should I hook up with him?" Brunette asked from the stall.

"Yeah," her friend replied, touching up her lipstick. "He's hot."

"But he has a girlfriend . . . and a fiancée."

Blonde paused as she tied her hair back in a ponytail. "Well, they aren't here, are they?"

Brunette emerged from the stall, smiling. "Well, no . . ."

So here was another reason girls drink until they pass out or give a blow job to a stud muffin who is engaged: It gives them a story to tell their girlfriends and keeps them feeling connected to the people who count.

Nicole acknowledged the latter in a conversation we had in late winter.

"I'd like to go to the gym on Saturdays instead of lying in bed hung over. But if I didn't go drinking, my friends would get mad. I don't want to lose them over it."

And if she chose a treadmill over Patty or Ann, everyone would know instantly, just as everyone knew within twenty-four hours of the night that Patty had hooked up with Curly Blond. Maybe they read an instant message, or IM, about it or heard someone talking in the food court. Maybe someone who took history with Patty passed it along to a classmate in chemistry. As one GW student told me, "In the hookup culture, a night of dirty fun is not a private affair." Such public gossip mattered less to Patty than it might have, however, because she had Nicole to console her.

While these friendships can fade with time, many continue well past college. Exhibit A: HBO's *Sex and the City*, which college women still watch in syndication since it went off the air in 2004 and consistently rate among their favorite shows. The number one reason for its lasting appeal is not the four stars' wardrobes or even their unreserved, occasionally kinky, sex; it is the relationship among Carrie, Miranda, Charlotte and Samantha. Independent careerists all, they depended on each other. Mr. Big, Carrie's love, summed this up in the final episode when he said to Carrie's friends: "You are her three loves. A guy would be lucky to come in fourth."

One night at Shooters, the cowboy bar in Durham popular with Duke students, the disk jockey put on Cyndi Lauper's 1980s hit "Girls Just Want to Have Fun." Immediately, the dance floor swarmed with young women dancing, grinning and singing together, their bare arms waving in the smoky air. The next tune, a hip-hop classic called "The Grind Date," brought out the boys. Girls partnered with them, facing away. The girls' behinds moved in sync with their partners' frontsides: "dry sex," some call it, or "freakin'," the naughty child of a previous generation's Twist, Jerk and Frug. The guys' eyes were glued to their partners' body parts, but the girls' eyes were on each other and their smiles were for each other.

. . .

Of course, many girls in college make and keep good guy friends. But they also begin to see guys in general either as adversaries or, at best, as fools. In the unhooked culture, friends can easily turn into "fuckbuddies," which can change or even destroy the original friendship. The age-old questions of whether friends make good lovers, or lovers can end up as good friends—memorialized in movies such as *When Harry Met Sally* in 1989 and *Annie Hall* twelve years earlier—are even harder for this generation to answer.

Nicole and Patty talked about this with some regret.

"It's very hard to let down your guard when a guy is being nice and appears to not be trying to get in your pants," Nicole said.

Patty agreed. "We're not friends with guys at GW. If you're not hooking up with them, they're not your friends."

She continued, "Everything is so casual here. I've kissed a lot of boys but never been to a movie with one or to dinner. I want a cute guy who enjoys me as much as my friends enjoy me."

Nicole was little comfort.

"It will never happen in college," she said. "Guys here are stupid. That's why I can kiss them."

The weekend after this conversation, Nicole took Patty as her date to her sorority's semiformal dance on a large, open-air boat that cruised the Potomac River in sight of Washington's splendid, well-lighted monuments. Nate, her current hookup buddy, was unavailable, and she figured if she had asked another guy, he would expect to hook up at the end of the night.

OLD-FASHIONED COURTSHIP

Shortly after that cruise, Nicole did find a cute guy who appeared to genuinely like her. His name was Michael, he was twenty-four, a medical student in Dallas and the youngest son in a wealthy Greek family. She had met him at a party the summer before her sophomore year. They had talked about her plans for medical school and e-mailed each other during fall semester. When she came home for winter break, she telephoned and left a message on his answering machine. He called back and asked if he could pick her up the next night. He arrived at the front door at exactly nine p.m., the time they had agreed upon. They drove to a bar, where they chatted about school in that sort of inconsequential way people do when they're first getting to know each other. Later he said, "Let's go get a coffee and something to eat."

At Café Brazil, a hip hangout in Dallas known for its quesadillas and cheesecake, they turned to more personal topics such as family, and barely touched their food. Michael revealed that his dad had been at the World Trade Center during the terrorist attack of September 11, 2001, and escaped unharmed. "I've never felt so comfortable talking to someone before," he told her.

Nicole felt pleased—and nervous. At ease being the pursuer, she wasn't sure how to feel about being pursued. He's brilliant, she thought. He's a second-year medical student. No way is he interested in me.

But he was. About two a.m., as he drove her home, Michael asked about her plans for New Year's Eve.

"I don't have any," she replied.

They discussed this as he walked her to the front door. He didn't believe her. "You're twenty years old and you don't have any plans? You want to come with me and my friends to Las Vegas?"

Whoa, thought Nicole. What's going on here? It wasn't clear what surprised her most—his generous invitation or his courtly behavior that night, which certainly wasn't like anything she had enjoyed in college.

Nicole's mother, Daphne, gave her permission to fly to Las Vegas, but not without qualms. What if it did turn serious? Like many upper-middle-class parents, she viewed boyfriends as a dangerous distraction from college studies. Nicole had admitted to me earlier in the year that she took her mother's caution to heart: "It affects me a lot. I know how hard she's worked to get me to college, and I wouldn't want to let her down."

Daphne had grown up in Texas, the daughter of an advertising executive and a homemaker. A fiery girl herself, she dated on and off in high school, resenting mightily the southern tradition that said good girls didn't go out on weekends unless invited by boys. She met Niko on a trip to Greece when she was in college, but when he suggested they get married, she declined. She enrolled in a university in Ohio and earned a law degree. She didn't, as she put it, "deprive myself of male companionship" in college, but she also didn't get serious with anyone. After law school, she married Niko and joined a Dallas law firm.

She had never known quite what to say to her daughters about love—either her love for their father or the concept itself. She had felt love's pull many years earlier, during the tumultuous nine-year courtship between two continents with the man who would become her husband. Five years into their relationship, she and Niko had had what she called a "bloody breakup," and she had been ready to burn the dozens of letters he had written when her mother stopped her. "You have evidence that someone once loved you very much," her mother said. "Save the letters for your children."

So she did. But her marriage had not been easy. When the girls started showing interest in boys, she read with them Longfellow's narrative of *Evangeline* and Shakespeare's *Romeo and Juliet*—tales of devotion and doom. "Love moderately," she advised them.

Nicole and her sister, Cleo, had picked up on the tension between their parents, as most children do. Of the marriage, Nicole had told me, "I don't ever hear my mom and dad say 'I love you.' I don't want to end up like that."

Nicole considered Michael's invitation the day following their date.

He wasn't just another guy she was interested in hooking up with. He had looks, intelligence and class. She could see herself in a relationship with him—but at what cost to her independence? Her grades? Her friends? Her sanity? In her world, there was nothing like casual dating. You either hooked up with a guy or attached yourself to him. She called to decline, saying the airplane tickets were too expensive.

She wanted to be in love but didn't feel she could afford to be. Other girls I interviewed, such as Sienna and Mieka, wouldn't even admit they had any interest in love; hooking up had soured them to its possibilities. Heather Schell, an assistant professor of writing at GW, discovered this reluctance among her female students in a course she taught called "Love, American Style." The young women loved to discuss the chick-lit book *Bridget Jones's Diary* and the sexual follies of Jones and her horny boss, Daniel Cleaver. But they were not enthralled with *Jane Eyre* and Edward Rochester's lengthy courtship of Eyre. Quick flings were okay, but "love was rarely mentioned in our class discussions," she observed. "They were not that interested in it as a concept for their lives." Of all the readings she assigned, their favorite was an anthology of poetry called *The Hell with Love*. I was reminded, when she told me this, of something that Patty, Nicole's friend, had told me: "A lot of people's goals, though they won't admit it, is to have a great love. But they won't say it because it's the twenty-first century."

Barbara Dafoe Whitehead and David Popenoe, two scientists affiliated with the National Marriage Project at Rutgers University, saw this trend developing in the late 1990s. They surveyed unmarried Americans in their twenties about sex, love and marriage and found widespread cynicism about love, particularly among young women in their early twenties. They attributed these feelings in large part to the casual sex lives of their subjects.

Of course, young women's reluctance to give all for romantic love at this time in their lives is hardly irrational. Love is not an easy emotion for anyone to live with day after day, and for young women who work hard and play hard, it can embrace them in an almost paralyzing squeeze.

Anthropologist Fisher discovered its power by analyzing 2,500 brain scans from seventeen college students newly in love. The scans were taken of students looking at pictures of their new loves and pictures of mere acquaintances. Her team's initial findings, reported in her book *Why We Love*, are fascinating.

When students gazed on the faces of their beloveds, as opposed to acquaintances, their brains showed higher levels of activity in a section known as the caudate nucleus, a primitive area connected to basic functions such as eating and drinking as well as pleasure, motivation and focus. Similarly high levels of activity took place in the ventral tegmental area, which distributes the chemical dopamine to various regions of the brain, including the caudate nucleus. Dopamine spurs the release of testosterone, the lust hormone. It can increase attentiveness but also sleeplessness, loss of appetite and dependency.

"No wonder lovers talk all night or walk till dawn, write extravagant poetry and self-revealing e-mails, cross continents or oceans to hug for just a weekend," Fisher writes. "Drenched in chemicals that bestow focus, stamina and vigor, and driven by the motivating engine of the brain, lovers succumb to a Herculean courting urge."

When one partner rejects another, some of these same chemicals reappear in force, Fisher says, resulting in equally powerful emotions including hatred, rage and deep, deep sadness. Men are more likely than women to commit suicide after a breakup; women are more likely to become severely depressed.

Most young women don't know these specifics but they do recognize love as something serious, something that you don't win by being a contestant on a TV dating game or by sucking face with the Lothario on your hall. Loving someone deeply and with commitment is not about meeting only their own needs, their focus during this period of their lives, but someone else's needs as well. It is a mark of being an adult, and many of them don't think they're there yet. As one college senior put it, "Love is an old people's emotion."

FULL-SCALE ASSAULT

Undeterred by Nicole's refusal to fly to Las Vegas, Michael stepped up his campaign to win her affection.

He text-messaged her on her cell phone on New Year's Eve while she was at a bar with girlfriends, saying, "I wish you were here." When he returned, he called and suggested that they re-create the occasion in Dallas that coming Friday, exactly a week after the holiday. He then placed a call to her sister, Cleo, asking confidentially about Nicole's favorite things.

On Friday, he picked her up looking stunningly handsome in a dark suit and lavender shirt. She met him in a tea-length, bright red satin dress. They dined at an expensive Italian restaurant, barely touching their three courses but enjoying a bottle of cabernet. At one point, he slipped out of the dining room to call his roommate, and when they entered his apartment she realized why: The fireplace was lit, candles glowed from each step leading up to his second-floor loft and a photo of Times Square at midnight shone from the screen of his computer. White lilies, her favorite flower, peeked from every corner, chilled champagne and hand-painted chocolates waited for her on a table. He excused himself to go to the kitchen.

She followed him moments later and found him preparing hot chocolate. Later, they piled blankets and gelato, her favorite dessert, along with the hot chocolate into the back of his SUV and headed for the countryside. He popped in a CD and as it played, Nicole realized he had made it himself, burning "Kodachrome," "Cecilia," and other songs that were her favorites. He had planned to drive to his family's retreat house, but it was late so they parked in a field instead. She popped a chocolate in her mouth and as she did so, he took her chin and gently kissed her. "My intention," he reassured her, "was not to get you in the back of my car." They cuddled and made out until four a.m.

He took her home, and only a few hours later called to ask her to brunch. After brunch, he dropped her back at her house and she went straight to her bedroom upstairs. The little things he had done on that date, he didn't have to do them. He could have gotten her into the SUV without them. But the fact that he went to the trouble of finding out she liked not just flowers but lilies, not just Paul Simon but "Kodachrome," such attention to detail overwhelmed her. This was the way she had heard that men used to woo women, but it was completely foreign to her.

She sat down on her bed and burst into tears. The emotional wall she had built over a year and a half at school to keep attachment at bay was crumbling one bonbon at a time.

Once back at school with her battlefield buddies, she got a grip on her feelings. She told herself that the distance between herself and Michael would allow her to get to know him slowly, over the phone and in e-mails. "I'm not against a relationship," she said, a big change for her. "But I'm against a relationship that would consume all of my time."

Three weeks later, during spring break, she took off for Acapulco with Patty and four other girlfriends. Michael had encouraged her to go, saying, "That's the kind of experience you need to have in college." Early one evening she and a couple of girlfriends, out for a stroll with several guys they had met, took off their blouses and started running down a street until the guys yelled at them to put their tops back on. On another evening, she exchanged a few kisses for bead necklaces with guys in a bar—a common stunt in college. But unlike Patty and the other girlfriends, she hooked up with no one.

"I didn't want to cheat on Michael for some half-naked boys," she said.

Shortly after her return, in late April, Nicole flew to Dallas and stayed with Michael over the weekend. Michael talked about his last girlfriend, the first woman he had had sex with. She told him about having sex with James, of how they had always done it in the dark and how quickly it was over. He was appalled at James's selfishness, at how little James had done to give her pleasure. Eventually, he made love to her, tenderly and with the lights on.

She told me this story upon her return over dinner with her friend Patty. I asked her whether she felt cherished—a word that conveys respect, commitment, playing for keeps.

"I don't like the word 'cherish,' " she said. "It sounds like someone is putting you up on a shelf. I want to crave someone and be craved in return. Michael and I crave each other." She was obviously still in that first, fabulously lustful stage of a relationship—but also moving into love and a feeling of ownership. She continued, comparing her last real boyfriend, William, to Michael.

"William was a rush to the head, a tumble in the grass. I will always love him. With Michael, it's more realistic and somehow bigger. We talk about what we're going to do in the future, how to incorporate family life into our career plans. I like being in a relationship where he's all mine."

Patty had never had a guy fall hard for her or, to use that old-fashioned expression, court her. Nor did she know any girls who had. Listening to her friend, she shook her head, concerned.

"Dear Lord" is all she could think of to say.

Sometimes Nicole would wake up in the middle of the night feeling Michael's love wrapped around her like a light blanket. But one night she awoke out of a nightmare in which she had found out she was pregnant and Michael, on hearing the news, had run away. She lay awake for an hour, thinking. The baby, she reasoned, represented her strong feelings for Michael. His departure signaled her plans to study abroad for the summer.

Beginning in late May, she would be in Greece, shadowing a hospital physician. A month after that, she'd be in Spain studying Spanish literature. Michael would be entering his third year of medical school, making rounds in the hospital and being on call twenty-four hours a day. Serious college relationships last, on average, twelve to eighteen months. They had had only four months and were separated for most of that time. Soon they would be living intense, rich lives thousands of miles apart. What chance did their relationship have to survive?

We discussed this on Greek Easter weekend. Every year, her parents host an Easter Sunday celebration for forty or fifty people at their house. Her father and his pals roast a lamb over a fire, starting early in the morning, and by early afternoon guests start arriving for hours of feasting, gossiping and drinking.

This year, Daphne had invited both William's and Michael's families. Nicole flew down, and a day later, so did Cleo. As Cleo and I sat beside the family pool on Friday afternoon, Nicole slipped in through the back gate, greeting us in a sleeveless white blouse, ruffly black skirt and Burberry-plaid flats she had borrowed from her mother's closet. "Michael's short," she said, needing, for some reason, to explain the shoes. Just back from spending the night at Michael's apartment, she was radiant. She gave me a tour of her room: her white antique bed, dresser and chest of drawers, the dozens of photos of her high school girlfriends, pom-poms from school basketball games and lacrosse matches. When she was in eighth grade, she told me casually, Michael was a senior at the boys' school that partnered with her school. Did I want to see a photo she had taken of the two of them with her digital camera?

Suddenly, she went from perky to pensive. "Michael is so serious," she said. "I still have a couple of years before I have to be serious and substantial. I want to be with him—but across the ocean? How is that going to work?"

Distance is the third partner in the relationships of many girls this age—making connections easier to sustain for some girls like Jamie, but more difficult for other girls. I asked Nicole if the relationship was worth waiting for.

"You just have to have faith it will work out," she answered. "But it's so, so hard. It hurts so much. I've cried so many times. You put names on each other—boyfriend, girlfriend—but it doesn't feel any better." Her admission was a moving reminder of how tender young women can be underneath their tough-girl posture.

Cleo, listening, commiserated. "Women have so many options," she said, "and yet we never have the time to figure out which one is best."

Nicole continued, "When I'm home, Michael and I spend all of our time together. He's worth it. But it's so frustrating, *truly*. We're both about leading our lives without affecting the other person. Sometimes I ask myself, Should I end it?"

In truth she saw herself as a kind of Sara Thomas figure in her favorite movie, *Serendipity,* a girl who turns down her first real love, convinced that one day she and he will reunite—which, in Hollywood, they do.

She never got that chance.

During the Easter celebration the next day, Michael hardly spoke to her. At first she couldn't figure out why. Was it because his parents were there? Or the presence of her old boyfriend, William? By early evening, she was getting the feeling that something was wrong. Finally, he got up to go, gave her a hug and said, "Well, goodbye."

He said he had exams to study for. She was leaving for Washington the next day and then, in another month, to Europe. And all he had to say was, "Well, goodbye"?

She text-messaged him later on her cell phone: "I'd like to say a proper goodbye tonight. Maybe a coffee break?"

He replied, "I really don't know what else there is to say."

A few weeks earlier, she had told me that both she and Michael were "adamant" about being able to pursue their separate career dreams without it affecting their relationship. She was able to. He, apparently, was not.

When she called him later, he told her, "I can't do this long distance anymore. I can't be with someone only once a month." He feared he was holding her back from having lots of experiences, and she suspected he also was afraid that she might cheat on him during their time apart.

His last girlfriend had cheated on him after they had been together more than a year, his cousin had told Nicole. Even a casual hookup on Nicole's part would break his heart. This, then, is one result of the unhooked culture on guys: It increases their fear of commitment because, like girls, they can never be sure when they're going to be disconnected. If a relationship has any problems at all—such as hundreds, even thousands, of miles between the pair—it may not be worth pursuing.

In high school, hooking up is adopted as the cool thing to do. In fact, you have to do it to some extent even if what you really want is a boyfriend, as Anna did. If you don't hook up, you're considered weird. The only cautionary voices girls hear—and only some girls at that—come from their parents. Sienna's mother, Beth, kept up a running conversation with Sienna not only about the perils of hooking up but the possibilities to be found in a serious relationship. Anna's mother shared with Anna the highs and lows of her dating years. Both mothers gave their daughters increasing latitude to make their own decisions—Anna's mom more than Sienna's—but their steady chatter forced these sophomores to continually reflect on what they and their classmates were doing. Mieka's mother, unfortunately, did not feel comfortable talking with Mieka about issues of intimacy other than to tell her not to have sex. Simple admonitions like that cannot compete with the other, louder voices of the unhooked culture—voices whose volume only increases once girls get to college.

Hooking up in college may be no more than sampling the goods away from the watchful eyes of your parents—"a fun time had by all." But as Nicole and her friends experienced, it also can morph into a serious power struggle between the sexes, fueled by booze and souring girls on guys and guys on girls. Nicole was a young woman of strong temperament—and this helped her survive the ups and downs of campus social life better than many women might. But when she found a young man who loved her and whom she loved, she discovered how hard trust was to come by in the unhooked culture. Without that trust, the odds of making a relationship work were slim.

When, on that Easter weekend, Michael expressed reservations about continuing their relationship, it wasn't clear to Nicole whether he had just pressed the "Pause" button or punched "Stop." Had she just been a rebound girl? The ambiguity was killing her.

Nicole was the kind of girl—and there are millions of others—who wanted an assertive partner who spoke his mind as she did. Michael really wasn't that guy. "He was so passive," she complained later. She had suffered through a muddy relationship with William, but that seemed different somehow, more innocent, perhaps because she had never had sex with William. The physical, as well as emotional, intimacy she and Michael had shared attached her to him in a way she hadn't foreseen.

"At first I was the cautious one. Then I took the bait. It all seems tainted now," she would say later.

She had never fought to keep a relationship going and wasn't about to start. Apparently he wasn't, either. Patience and the willingness to work through difficulties do not come easily to a Google generation that expects problems to be quickly resolved. In the weeks that followed Easter Sunday, the two of them exchanged words, but it was unclear whether they desired to restore what they had had or simply get back at each other.

They messaged on their phones and computer several times a day for a couple of weeks after she left Dallas.

"I had hoped it wouldn't turn out this way," he wrote.

"I didn't ask you to start this," she replied.

"Nicole, I'm going into the third year of medical school. People get divorced in the third year," he wrote.

"I'm upset that you've completely shut me off without any warning," she replied. "Remember all that stuff you did for me after New Year's? What was that about?"

"I wanted to do something nice for you," he replied.

And so it went as she studied in the library for her finals at GW in genetics, cellular biology and physics. Her grades in a couple of subjects were not what they should be for an aspiring medical student, and she needed to ace the finals. At the same time, she couldn't help but continue her war of words with Michael. She and Michael were tormented by the omnipresence of technology, captives in a way previous generations never were. Michael's number would appear on her cell phone screen and she wouldn't answer his call. He would text-message her: "Would you please pick up or call me?" She would call and he would ignore her call.

"I know what you're doing and I'm not impressed," she told him in one message.

Meanwhile, William e-mailed her that he had seen Michael at a golf tournament in deep conversation with a young woman. That night, Nicole grabbed Patty and headed for Daedalus, a Washington watering hole she liked. She had heard that her old buddy Nate was going to be there, and former hookup partners could usually be persuaded to do a little consoling.

She danced and flirted with Nate. They kissed and took a taxi back to his room. She lay down with him on the bed, put her head on his chest and fell asleep, as comfortable as if she were a drowsy little girl again, in her own bed at home.

"I don't want to go back to the hookup culture," she told me the next day. "For one thing, it's dangerous. One friend I know slept with a guy in Europe and got chlamydia, gonorrhea and genital warts all from that one guy. I was the one she confided in.

"Hooking up is also very selfish," she went on. "It's all about what you want, not what the other person wants."

But she also didn't feel like "putting myself out there again for a guy who will give me bullshit."

"Maybe I'm too young for love," she concluded. "Maybe I should just stick with the girls, go out with them and laugh later at all the stupid things we did." Two weeks later she was on a plane to Athens.

section three

How We Got There

Culture, as defined by *Webster's New World College Dictionary*, means "the ideas, customs, skills and arts of a people or group that are passed along to succeeding generations." Sometimes this "passing along" is done intentionally and with forethought, as when Sienna's mother, Beth, told tales of her own dating, hoping Sienna would see the value in taking time to get to know a boy before she decided to hook up with him.

Often, however, adults pass on ways of thinking and being without knowing that they do so. Their children absorb these habits of the mind and heart and then interpret them in their own way, influenced by their own experiences. This is how the unhooked culture came to be and, quite frankly, why it's so difficult to explain. I wish I could tell you, as some people will, that hooking up is the result of a hypersexualized media, or rapacious commercial interests, or parents who don't spend much time with their kids once those kids become teenagers. It is a bit of all three of those things and a bit of many others. I have chosen three of the others to write about—three developments in our culture over the last several decades whose influences surfaced over and over during the year that I spent with my young women. Considered together, they do not explain everything. But they explain a lot.

Feminism

SHAIDA'S STORY

"Within a male-dominated sexual campus, take the term
'hooking up' and make it your own."
—SHAIDA, NINETEEN

L ess than ten minutes after she arrived at Shooters Saloon in downtown Durham, Shaida was dancing on a platform in a black tube top,
short black skirt and black stilettos.

Behind her, a larger-than-life-sized white plastic stallion balanced on
its hind legs, and two giant video screens played old Western movies. To
her left, a bosomy blonde was bouncing on the saddle of a mechanical
bull. Below and to her right, a few feet away on a wooden dance floor, a
blond guy with a beer bottle in his mouth was gyrating between two girls.

I had just arrived. Wanting to get a view of the crowd, I started climbing a set of stairs leading to the second floor. As I reached the top, I
froze. Less than ten feet away, a waif in a purple halter top and shorts was
pulling a boy on top of her and a pool table. Should I walk by and pretend I hadn't noticed, or return downstairs? The girl glanced over at
me, then got back to the business at hand, so I stayed.

A balcony ran the full length of the second floor, and from there I
could watch Shaida moving her torso to music in a way I didn't think was

humanly possible. It dawned on me that hardly anyone else was paying attention to her. Later I realized that that was because they knew her already.

Shaida was a sophomore at Duke who, a little over a year earlier, as a freshman, wrote this in the campus newspaper, *The Chronicle*:

> I have a different kind of proposition for the women of Duke: Lose the pearls and get the La Perla. . . . Ask for more when he's done and you're still going. Within a male-dominated sexual campus, take the term "hooking up" and make it your own. Ask a guy to a semiformal because of the simple fact that every time you pass him in the Bryan Center you think, "Damn, I'd like to beat that."

And this:

> There is too much of a gap at Duke between the woman who knows what she wants and the foolish girl who doesn't know what she is. . . . Really, Ladies, instead of prematurely placing a claim on the disinterested boy toy, we should focus a little more on empowering and placing a claim on ourselves.

She also wrote about racial tensions on campus and the Israeli–Palestinian conflict. But her columns about sex, gender and power were what made her famous or, in some students' minds, infamous. Duke, true to its southern roots, was a campus that was highly ambivalent about how powerful young women should be in all areas of life, including the bedroom. Shaida, a bronze-skinned, black-haired Persian with a stud in her right nostril, arrived from California with a partial answer: A strong woman who desired a particular man should, provided he was willing, be able to take that man to bed and do whatever she damn well pleased.

She didn't have to love him or even know him very well. If she couldn't do this, she wasn't really empowered, no matter how good her grades were or which sorority she belonged to.

Her prose wouldn't have raised eyebrows on any number of campuses now, where student magazines feature photos of students in the buff and first-person accounts of sex with strangers. But at Duke, Shaida drew the kind of reaction feminist writer Naomi Wolf received from one critic for her 1997 book *Promiscuities*: "Go ahead and do it, but for God's sake don't write about it." As Jamie had found during her awful freshman year at Duke, plenty of young women there were doing what Shaida wrote about, but they didn't talk about it publicly or, God forbid, openly admit that they liked it.

I had been introduced to Shaida at Duke's Women's Center in the early afternoon preceding our visit to Shooters. A cozy set of offices on the main West Campus, with a comfortable lounge and feminist magazines ranging from *Ms.* to *Bitch*, the center was one of the few places on campus Shaida felt comfortable expressing her opinions. We talked briefly and made arrangements for me to pick her up the next night at eleven to go to Shooters.

Although under age, Shaida had no trouble getting into the club, located in a grimy part of town. She was a regular patron, friendly with the owner and the disk jockey. She introduced me to some of her friends, who were sitting off to the side, then headed toward the table and for the next few hours, alternated between dancing—either alone or with a partner—and chatting with her pals.

At about two-thirty a.m., I started searching for her to tell her I was ready to go. A girlfriend said she had already left. I would later learn that she didn't leave alone. It was a decision that, along with several others, she would come to regret over our year together as she struggled to figure out the possibilities and limitations of her sexual power.

. . .

Feminism is undeniably a driving force behind the phenomenon of hooking up. What it should say about sex and relationships has been a matter of debate since the birth of the modern movement in the 1960s and 1970s. Women's liberation back then meant, among many other things, being free to have a sexual appetite and act on it with as much abandon as women assumed men did. Sex—in or outside a relationship—was as natural and healthy as breast milk. With the help of the newly available birth control pill and loosened abortion laws, college students exchanged partners, and so did their parents. Young women followed rock stars, teachers took their students to bed and the phrase "sleeping around" came into use. The women and men who engaged in "free love" were actually fairly small in number, but they attracted so much media attention that they came to define the era in the minds of many Americans.

In earlier decades, a woman's worth had been determined by finding a husband to love. By the '70s, the most visible leaders of the women's movement were saying that loving yourself was the preferred goal. Marriage equaled slavery; loving another equaled bondage; and flirting equaled game-playing. Wanting a man for anything other than pleasure meant that you had sold out to the patriarchal culture.

Feminists such as Betty Friedan and Gloria Steinem made Americans aware of the sexual double standard and gave women permission to rethink what they wanted out of sex and relationships, including marriage—healthy developments, on the whole. They also drew needed attention to demeaning portrayals of women in the media and the prevalence of sexual and domestic violence.

But feminists have never spoken with one voice. By the early 1980s, new voices had emerged, some of whom said the earlier position on sex was too extreme. Power in one's private life did not necessarily have to look like power in public life; sexual experimentation was valuable but in the context of meaningful, mutually respectful and, yes, loving relationships. These women weren't as well-known as their predecessors and may not always have acted according to their rhetoric, but they articulated standards that forced women and men to think about their desires and behavior.

Shaida, the year I observed her, was a throwback to the late 1960s. So were a number of other young women I met, including those who rejected the idea of having anything to do with feminism. These young women saw themselves as freely sexual beings privately and publicly. They bared their breasts in low-cut tops—not all that different from burning your bra if you think about it. They took young men to bed and then, like Nicole at GW, dumped them. At our first meeting at the Women's Center, Shaida said to me, "I can differentiate between the men I like and the men I use—and I do use them."

What I also was hearing from some of these women privately, however—Nicole and Anna, for example—was that they hoped to find someone to love who would love them back. When they raised this with other young women, they said, they sometimes got laughed at. Lynn Harris, a writer in her twenties, talked about this in an article she wrote for *Glamour* magazine. "We're supposed to be all 'I'm a strong woman, and I'm fine on my own!' " she wrote. "I know a six-letter word for 'Greek god of dancing'!"

She continued, "When we cop to being lonely, we're seen as that sad girl in the misty video. Or worse, we hear—as I did, right to my single face—that wanting a man is selling out to The Man, some sort of unholy alliance between the patriarchy and Lifetime TV."

Harris didn't buy this and evoked Norah Jones, the popular, syrupy, Grammy-winning singer-songwriter. "Let's face it: The desire to feel truly, goopily, cozily in love is, hello, human. Norahjonesing is not caving; it's living."

FEELING DIFFERENT

The planned community of Irvine, California, sits in the flat middle of Orange County, its stucco homes having replaced strawberry fields only thirty years ago. Shaida grew up in Irvine, and it was at Northwood High School, among 2,000 well-to-do white and Asian students, that she first learned how hard it is to feel powerful when what you mostly feel is different.

Her father, Hesam, who had come to this country from Iran as a young man, sold the luxury cars that Irvine's wealthier kids drove. Her mother, Nasim, also an Iranian immigrant, worked for the state highway department, unlike other mothers who regularly took the spa at Palm Springs. Shaida's body was curvaceous, not reed-thin like the classmates she called the "it" girls, as in "They think they are *it*." One afternoon she showed me photos of these cookie-cutter cuties in her high school yearbook: three full pages of the same ten seniors, all blonde, all in bikinis, sports attire or strapless gowns, all standing next to pools and tennis courts and BMWs.

Children who feel uncomfortably unlike their classmates react in a variety of ways. Some try to disappear into the crowd, making themselves so much like everyone else that no one will see them. Some find refuge in organizations in which they can be themselves but disappear again when they move outside those safety zones. Some think of themselves in positive terms and claim any environment as their own. And some, including Shaida, decide to be so in-your-face different that people have to pay attention to them. Not particularly comfortable in their skin, they take pleasure in discomforting others.

In her junior year at Northwood High, Shaida began making a conscious effort to make a name for herself. By senior year, she was president of five clubs, an outspoken editor on the school newspaper, a member of the dance team and founder of a students' rights organization to support gays and lesbians. Her biggest supporter was her mother. Nasim had been raised in Tehran by a father who encouraged her independence and a mother who, joined to a man in an arranged marriage at thirteen, wanted a different life for her daughter. Nasim had moved to California by herself at eighteen and worked her way through college, acquiring a bachelor's degree in engineering. She wanted nothing to do with an arranged marriage but was uncomfortable with the idea of marrying outside her culture. Shortly after she met Hesam, she married him and then gave birth to Shaida and later two boys, working all the while.

In Shaida's senior yearbook, Nasim wrote to her oldest child, "Never stop fighting. Never stop expressing yourself. Never stop being Shaida." At Duke, Shaida took the words to heart, though for a cause that made her mother uncomfortable: female sexuality. As she had in high school, Shaida would step outside the boundaries of what was considered proper partly so she wouldn't have to compare herself to anyone else.

As soon as she arrived at Duke, she had recognized that hooking up was the main social event on campus, promoted by a handful of elite fraternities and sororities that, along with a couple of sports teams, ran Duke's social life. The irony didn't escape her: She had gone from a high school of stereotypes to a college of stereotypes. At Duke, though, young women seemed a bit more—well, she wasn't quite sure what the word was. Old-fashioned? Desperate? Their game seemed to be solely about attracting men. In her view, everything they did, they did for men rather than for themselves, and they didn't even think about what that might mean for their long-term happiness.

She decided to play the sex kitten to force a public debate over the fine line between being the subject of one's life and the object of someone else's. She hadn't hooked up that much in high school, but found that being flirtatious came easily to her. As a freshman, she had an almost endless supply of partners to choose from. She went for the types who had rarely given her the time of day in Irvine: a lacrosse player, a football player, several fraternity guys. With each one, she stopped before intercourse. Sex, in any form, would be on her terms.

She took on sorority girls in the newspaper because, in her mind, they played into the woman-as-object stereotype. She wrote, for example, about a lip-sync contest at Shooters, sponsored by the Sigma Chi fraternity, in which sorority members competed by dancing on tables in their underwear, garter belts, fishnet stockings and bras. The winning act was also the most outrageous, in Shaida's view: Sorority sisters squirted whipped cream on each other and then licked it off while guys cheered and clapped. Was this empowerment? she wondered.

"Sorority women who dance on tables, take a man home on their own terms and carry themselves—at a bar and in the classroom—with a sense of self-worth have my respect," she wrote. "Sorostitutes who lick whipped cream off one another to visually appease men do not." Neither, she wrote in the same column, do sorority sisters who allow guys from certain fraternities to take them to bed in order to boost a sorority's social standing.

She received support for her views from people like Donna Lisker, director of Duke's Women's Center, who told me that "one of the things that makes me the saddest is that these incredibly smart women are performing for the men. They think they're free agents and don't see the cultural pressures they're caving in to." But students didn't much like what Shaida had to say. *The Chronicle* was bombarded by letters to the editor. Not much difference between dancing on a table as you do and licking whipped cream off a girlfriend, one writer said. Another young woman asked, "So sleeping around is acceptable when done as part of some misguided feminist agenda, but unacceptable when done for the purposes of campus social climbing?"

. . .

Perhaps one of the reasons Shaida took on the issue of gender equality and sexual power when she got to Duke was that in her own Iranian culture, women have little of either. Married Muslim women are, by custom and law, expected to be subordinate to their husbands and their husbands' families in virtually every respect, including the raising of children. Even today in Iran, many marriages are arranged, financial payments are promised to the bride's family and the bride is expected to be a virgin. If she's not, no money is forthcoming.

Officially, sex in Iran is primarily meant for producing children. Images of nude or nearly nude women are available on satellite television, but little attention is given to the emotional aspects of sex and marriage, and what there is focuses almost solely on the wife's feelings for her husband. A wife is expected to feel attached to her husband and to show her devotion daily, but a husband is not supposed to be too enamored of his wife lest he seem to have lost control over her.

Shaida had seen her mother, Nasim, an outwardly independent woman, struggle with these expectations. She also knew that her grandmother, whom she called Momonjoon, believed in them. Momonjoon, who moved in with the family after Shaida's grandfather died, wore traditional Muslim dress, including the *roosaree*, or scarf, and spoke only Farsi. Every morning at five, she rose to read the Koran, her finger running over each line, her lips moving silently in prayer. She walked Shaida and, later, Shaida's brothers to elementary school and greeted them when they came home with bowls of dates and pastries and a pot of hot tea. Although Shaida rarely talked to her about social life, her presence was a daily reminder of what Shaida felt she had to somehow overcome.

Beginning in the second semester of her freshman year, Shaida began considering the value of two-way, emotionally intimate relationships. She tried setting up a dating service on campus, which flopped for lack of interest. She designed and co-taught a course on the hookup culture called "Dating and Mating" and even that, despite her best efforts to keep discussions focused on lasting relationships, turned into a course on hooking up.

It was in that course that she met Tomas. He was a senior and a lean, dark-haired artist. One night he asked her out to dinner. "Don't be a seductress," he told her. "Just be yourself. That's much sexier." She fell in love despite herself.

They started hanging out together. Within a month, he asked her to move into his off-campus house, and she did. They cooked dinner together almost every night and washed each other's laundry. She trimmed his eyebrows. When they had sex for the first time—her first, but not his—she was in so much pain that he took her, the next day, to the doctor's office. She sent him a greeting card saying, "I'm glad you were my first"; a sign of the times if there ever was one.

Shaida and Tomas began making a life together, adjusting their schedules accordingly. He'd listen to her problems; she would accompany him to job interviews to calm his nervousness. After a couple of months they started calling each other girlfriend and boyfriend, though only to close friends. "At Duke, you can't be too open about real relationships," she told me.

In the summer after her freshman year, shortly before I met her, Tomas flew out to Orange County to visit her, at her expense. He went with her to buy a white Pomeranian puppy, and they named it Persia. He then flew to Chicago, where he had gotten a job, hoping to be a model and making no promises. She realized that their relationship was over and that maybe, given their different points in life, that was okay. But one thing bothered her: He had told her he loved her in Spanish but never in English. In a letter, she asked why.

He responded in August by sending her a scrapbook for her birthday, a professional-looking binder filled with old e-mails and ticket stubs, organized chronologically—by friendship, courtship, romance—and ending with this line:

"I'm sorry I never loved you. I didn't know if I ever would."

The next day she flew to Miami to visit friends and ended up getting drunk and stoned and making out with a friend of one of her guy pals.

BACK ON THE MARKET

Psychologists suggest that there are three parts to the kind of emotional intimacy Shaida sought. The first is attachment that becomes so deep you are willing to put your partner's well-being ahead of your own. The second is sharing interests, including some you might not have picked for yourself. The third is exchanging thoughts and feelings you would not tell anyone else. Shaida had experienced all of these with Tomas, as well as a fourth element: passion. In her view, nothing in life made sense without the anticipation that the earth was about to split open and swallow her and her lover. In this she was more Eastern than Western, following the scripts of ancient China and India that valued the female's carnal desires.

With Tomas out of the picture, and as her sophomore year began, she missed passion more than anything. So on that first weekend I met her, after she danced for a couple of hours at Shooters, she went back to her dorm room with a lacrosse player named Nathan who had pulled up her skirt while she was dancing. They had sex in her dorm room, she told me in an e-mail the next day, and she regretted it.

She described an incident that took place the night after the Nathan episode. At a campus diner, she had run into Jerome, another guy she had had her eye on, and he offered to walk her back to her dorm.

"What are you up to?" a friend of Jerome's asked him as the two headed out the door.

Jerome was nothing if not blunt: "I'm hitting on Shaida."

As they wandered across campus, making out every now and then, he asked her, "What are you looking for?"

"I just came out of a serious relationship," she responded. "I don't know. Just go with the flow, I guess."

She explained to him that she couldn't sexile her roommate for a second night in a row, so they went to his room in his fraternity house. As they started making out more heavily, she tried to get him to talk. ("Men get really annoyed when I do that," she told me later, "but I like the mind-body-soul connection. It's the way I look for intimacy during a hookup.")

"What are you thinking?" she asked him at one point.

"That you're really attractive," he said, then added, "I really want to have sex with you."

She helped him put on a condom and winced as he entered her. Then he surprised her.

"I'm sorry, this feels really wrong," he said. "I think of you more as a friend."

They stopped, she put her clothes on, he walked her back to her dorm and she went to bed disappointed again. She wasn't expecting Jerome, or any other guy, really, to fall in love with her right away. "But I thought at least I had my sexuality," she wrote in her e-mail. "Jerome blew that thought away."

Like Nicole, the GW sophomore who lured James to bed only to walk out on him after they had sex, Shaida was using her sexuality to feel something. But there was a difference. Nicole sought to feel avenged for James dumping her; Shaida wanted to feel prized for her desirability and skill. Nicole thought she had achieved her goal right after that infamous fall night but realized later that she wasn't completely over James. Shaida, too, felt like a failure as soon as she got back to her dorm room. Using sex as a means of boosting one's self-esteem can, and often does, backfire.

To her credit, Shaida was not one to sit around and mope. Over the next couple of weeks, in addition to going to classes in film, computer science and Arabic, she helped publicize a student conference on the Palestinian Solidarity Movement, drawing the ire of Jewish students by putting up a sign that read "Zionism = Ethnic Cleansing." She wrote a column accusing the campus police force of racism, and a humor essay about a conspiracy of squirrels to rid the campus of humans. As part of Breast Cancer Awareness Month, she and several girlfriends allowed female volunteers in the Women's Center to apply plaster of Paris to their naked torsos. When dried and removed, the busts were theirs to keep; Shalda placed hers, painted bright red, on the desk in her dorm room. "We need to take back our breasts," she was quoted as saying in a *Chronicle* article covering the event. "We see them as a man's tools and clearly they're not."

One afternoon, she ran into another political activist, Viktor, who said he wanted to talk to her. The previous year, he had approached her and admitted he wanted to date her even though he knew she only hooked up. She had told him that that wasn't true and gave him her phone number. Although they shared a couple of classes together after that, he had never raised the subject again, and as forward as she was, she wasn't forward enough to approach him. On this afternoon, he confessed that he still felt deeply about her. "If I fell in love with you, that would be it for me," he said.

That was her moment of power. She could make him work hard to get her, raising the chance that he'd work hard to keep her. That night, he stopped by to take her for a walk. Perhaps if this had been 1964 or even 1974, they would have made out, agreed to go out on another date and yet another, gradually becoming more intimate in body and mind. But on this autumn night, less than twelve hours after he first approached her on the quad, they ended up on the candy wrapper–strewn floor of a building on campus having intercourse. I confess I was shocked when she told me this, and could only conclude that the chemistry between them simply overpowered the self-control she thought she had.

"It was completely spontaneous," she wrote. "But it was intimate, relationship sex"—without the relationship, she neglected to add.

I had heard girls, like Anna's high school friend Jill, say that hooking up could lead to a relationship. But I had never witnessed it. For a brief while, I thought I would get that chance. Viktor wrote her the next day saying how great their experience had been. She wrote back, "It *was* wonderful. There's an intoxication that results from the bonding of the body and the soul . . . where sparks fly, colors blur and passion reigns supreme." A week later, they visited her dorm room, a sensuous cell with batik wall hangings and a burgundy shade covering the light fixture on the ceiling. They had sex again in her bed under a poster of Che Guevara.

"You are one of the most amazing people I've met," he told her that night.

He was not like the other guys she had known. He had little interest in sports and was planning a double major in public policy and Chinese. He didn't party and wouldn't be caught dead at Shooters. He didn't care if she had shaved her legs before they went out. And, most important, he was the first guy who would talk with her during sex, who called sex "making love" and who left her feeling that she had made love to a person and not just a man.

On the second night of their affair, he said two things that would haunt her in the days to come: "You'll make someone a great wife" and "I'm not a good person to love." She could tell he was pulling away from her, and was upset. Shortly before Thanksgiving, she wrote saying that she and Viktor had "kinda said goodbye." "Kinda," of course, because they had never actually been a couple. She had made the mistake of thinking that if the sex was great, they would move into a relationship.

I took Shaida out for breakfast on campus a few weeks after the Viktor saga came to a close. The fall term had ended, and her body sagged with exam fatigue and the stress that comes from multiple failed attempts at connecting intimately with another. She was looking for answers, and I had none. I knew that some theorists suggest that the quality of romantic relationships we have later in life is linked to the quality of our earliest attachments. So I asked about her childhood and her parents.

"My parents' relationship was never very stable and neither was their relationship to us," she began.

Nasim and Hesam fought over Hesam's family, who didn't like the independent woman he had married. They fought over money after Hesam started acquiring property and refused to put Nasim's name alongside his on the legal papers. They fought over Shaida, with Hesam accusing Nasim of spoiling Shaida and Nasim criticizing Hesam for not spending time with his daughter. These were loud, increasingly acrimonious fights resulting in recurring separations rather than compromises. Nasim moved herself and her children into a small house and sometimes, late at night, would slip into her daughter's bedroom and sing quietly to her sleeping child the Helen Reddy song "You and Me Against the World." As Shaida relayed such memories, I thought of Mieka, the high school girl whose father never lived with her. Both girls hungered for a lasting means of emotional support but didn't have much faith that men could provide it. Hooking up was a lousy replacement, but at least it was something over which they exercised some control.

Right before Shaida was to enter fifth grade, she and her brothers moved with Nasim to Tehran, where Nasim hoped to find peace away from her husband and his family. When Nasim discovered that she couldn't enroll Shaida in the American school there, however, they returned to Irvine. Shaida's most vivid memory of their quick departure from Iran was being told to leave her Barbie dolls behind, all fifty of them. She lived in six houses before she entered high school. Not only was her family life uncertain, but so was the bed in which she slept.

Shaida kept advising her mother to file for divorce, a difficult step for an Iranian woman to take no matter how strong-willed she is. Nasim finally divorced Hesam as Shaida started her senior year of high school, and Shaida watched the relationship between her parents gradually improve. On a visit I made to Nasim's home late in the year—a modern, airy house with hardwood floors and sharply angled doors and walls—Hesam and Nasim sat together in the family room and expressed regret that Shaida, the first of their three children, had had to suffer so many years of marital arguments. Like Nicole's Greek parents, they were a couple with strong opinions, freely expressed. But unlike Nicole's family, they had allowed their differences to become ugly and eventually split them up. Children can withstand divisions at home if they see those divisions worked on and resolved. Hesam and Nasim kept growing further and further apart. Hesam, in our interview, said he believed this helped explain some of Shaida's unhappiness at college.

More than his wife, he interpreted Shaida's sexual openness as an aggressive front to keep men from getting too close and possibly hurting her. He hoped that she would eventually tone herself down. "It will be difficult for someone to break through the barriers that are there," he said, "but if that happens, he will see that she is a beautiful person."

PUSHING THE LIMITS

In February, shortly after Duke students returned from winter break, the Blue Devils basketball team took on their fiercest rival, the University of North Carolina–Chapel Hill, at home. Hundreds of students had lived in tents on the lawn in front of the stadium—some for as long as a month—in order to acquire tickets for the big event. The day of the game, the students were still lounging around in what is affectionately known as Tent City, and every few minutes would burst into a cheer, "Go to hell, Carolina! Go to hell!"

Shaida was there, too, but screaming something else. Dressed in jeans and wearing a red bra over her T-shirt, she snaked her way through the crowd holding a placard and yelling, "Vagina! Vagina! Vagina!" Her job was to stir up interest for an event in the auditorium the next night: *The Vagina Monologues*. Occasionally, a smart-aleck male would bark back, "Why not Penis! Penis! Penis!"

Few works of entertainment have done more to encourage women to equate their sexuality with power than feminist playwright Eve Ensler's *Monologues*. First appearing off-Broadway in 1996, the Obie award–winning drama consists of a series of short ruminations with deliberately provocative titles such as "Reclaiming Cunt" and "He Liked to Look Down There." It includes a skit by an elderly woman seeking her own pleasure, and another on the rape of a thirteen-year-old girl. Ensler's message, which has played in theaters all over the world and claimed the attention of Glenn Close, Oprah Winfrey and other celebrities, is simple: Once women come to know and appreciate their vaginas and all that their vaginas can do, they will be less likely to allow men to abuse them and more likely to speak out against abuse.

Monologues enthusiasts tend to focus on either the knowing part of the message or the abuse part. The knowers say women are told from childhood that they shouldn't talk about their private parts. Public embarrassment around the word "vagina" makes girls believe that their bodies are dirty and that having sex is something good girls don't do or don't enjoy. If women are able to talk about vaginas, as well as menstruation, masturbation and orgasm, they lay claim to their desires and are better able to fulfill them. Given what I've heard young women say and do, they've gotten the message.

In interviews, Ensler always seemed more interested in her second point: that being ignorant about your body results in a feeling of powerlessness and encourages men to take advantage of you through rape, incest or genital mutilation. As her play picked up momentum on college campuses in particular, she hatched the idea of having it performed on or around Valentine's Day and using the phrase "V-Day" as a slogan for the bruises and scars of violence rather than the chocolates and roses of love. She was blasted by some for perpetrating a creed of victimization that one columnist called "positively criminal" and hailed by others as a cheerleader for women's rights. One member of the Duke cast, a senior, fell into the latter camp.

"*The Vagina Monologues* is not about lesbianism or man-hating," she wrote in the Duke *Chronicle*. "It's about grabbing our notoriously taboo sexuality by the horns and cultivating it. It's about liberation from the double standard. It's about saying what we feel. . . . And yes, it's about sex (gasp) and enjoying it."

Monologues ushered in a movement, fully ensconced on many campuses now, aimed at teaching young women how to enjoy sex. Sexual pleasure workshops are frequently sponsored by women's studies faculty. Some are for women only, and others, such as one at Washington University in St. Louis called "Good Vibrations: Women and Orgasms," are open to men as well. Sex-toy companies are invited to come to campus for show-and-tell. Although leaders at these events usually at least mention the emotions of sex and the obligations sex entails, their conversation for the most part focuses on the individual actor and her—or his—immediate pleasure. That the best sex is with someone you know well and love deeply takes a backseat to the means of achieving multiple orgasms.

On the night before the *Monologues* production, Shaida helped lead one of these workshops for women only. As I walked in, a counselor from the health center was explaining how a woman could receive pleasure from anal sex.

"It should never hurt, if done slowly and lovingly," she said. "But that's hard in college when you don't know how slow and loving your partner may be." She discussed how partners who wanted to use their fingers should wear "butt gloves" for hygienic reasons. In oral sex, dental dams should be used, she said. This elicited a few "fat chance" remarks.

An older woman named Tatiana, representing a company called

Temptations: Parties for Open-Minded Adults, then took the podium with a basket full of sexy edibles, massage tools and toys. She talked for a half-hour. I was about to conclude that this seminar would be confined to improving the mechanics of sex, when a third speaker stood up and asked the girls to name the characteristics they looked for in their partners.

"Patience," one girl said. The speaker wrote this answer on a blackboard. Other girls came forward: "Strength." "Nice to my friends." "A good listener." "A sense of humor." "Honesty." "Trust." "Someone who will treat me as an equal."

Finally, I thought, the group was going to get around to discussing something more than body parts. As Shaida realized, good sex—really good sex—demands the stimulation of the mind as well as the vagina. But it was not to be. Fewer than ten minutes had passed when the speaker announced that their time was over and asked for volunteers to clean up.

Shaida hurried over to her dorm room to check her e-mail before going to *Monologues* rehearsal. She pulled up a message from a freshman pledging the fraternity Alpha Epsilon Pi. The fraternity had given him a list of items to acquire that included a pair of Shaida's panties. Could she help him? She grimaced. Was a girl out there with her sexuality fair game for anybody? She guessed she knew the answer.

As she arrived at the Lesbian/Gay/Bisexual/Transgender Center for play practice, the girls in the show were preparing to block each scene one last time. While waiting for their directors to arrive, they discussed their parents' reactions to the provocative soliloquies they would perform the following night.

"My father doesn't want me to do it," one girl said. "My mother read the script and said it was interesting, but she doesn't think she will come."

"This is the most shocking thing I've ever done," another girl said.

"I keep telling my mom about it, and she's scandalized." A girl who identified herself as being from the Bible Belt said her parents supported her. "But my uncle and aunt live in a little town in South Carolina, and their pastor preached against the *Monologues* before it was performed at the local college." Another girl protested this: "I'm a devout Catholic. I think God would support this."

"One of my friends says that what we're saying is that women shouldn't get married and have children," another student said. "That's not it at all!"

The girls had more questions than answers, and they weren't the questions I was expecting. What is wrong with making a sexual experience the best it can be and, until it can be great, waiting to have it? Why, when a girl says she wants to be "in touch with her sexuality," do people assume she jumps into bed with every guy she meets? Couldn't she just as easily decide to stay a virgin?

"Your vagina is connected to your brain and your heart," said a girl named Victoria. "Don't we need to talk about that?"

The discussion underscored an impression that had been forming in my mind for several months: Young women could see their way out of the hookup habit if given the space and support to do so. Even Shaida spoke up briefly. "I used to be übersexualized," she said. "Now I'm more aware of the fact that the body is more than just a vagina."

Until that point, she had been uncharacteristically quiet. The play reminded her of the fact that she was deep into her version of a sophomore slump. She hadn't kissed a guy in more than three months. She couldn't muster up the energy to flirt or use her vibrator. She was also worried about her mother's reaction to what she planned for the next night.

She would not be alone onstage. Unlike the way the play is normally produced, with one solo monologue followed by another, the actresses in this production would group themselves around a speaker during her

performance and in some cases add to her soliloquy. (The scenes reminded me, in fact, of the candid, if coarse, discussions I had seen girls
having casually with each other at camp and other places.) Shaida suspected her mother would be uncomfortable with what her daughter did,
even if surrounded by friends.

Two hours before the play began that Saturday evening, Nasim and
Sara, Shaida's aunt, arrived to mark their seats in the front row. As soon
as the doors to Page Auditorium opened, they walked in, and soon the
thousand-seat hall was filled, about two-thirds with girls, as Salt-N-
Pepa sang over the sound system, "It ain't a man's world, no more
sugar and spice . . ."

Nasim had thought she was emotionally prepared for what she would
see that night. She had told herself that Shaida would be uncomfortable
saying some of the things she would have to say and doing some of the
things she'd have to do. An hour before the performance, she had swung
by a local grocery store and purchased a bouquet of assorted flowers to
give to Shaida after the play "to make her feel better."

But it was clear from the start that Shaida had little trouble acting her
parts. Early in the show, she and two other girls lay down on center stage.
When Shaida, in swishy black cropped pants and a bright yellow jacket,
spread her (clothed) legs apart and held a mirror up to her vagina, Nasim
gasped. Later, when in a short black nightgown, she put a pillow between her legs and started moaning, Nasim sank into her seat. "I'm not
sure I can stand this," she whispered to me.

Nasim had been raised in a Muslim family but was not a practicing
Muslim. Her daughter wasn't, either. But the old religious constraints
against women displaying their bodies in public still had a hold on Nasim.
This wasn't a question of whether or not Shaida should wear a burka; it
was whether she should pretend to get off in front of a thousand people.

"She goes beyond where she should," Nasim said, echoing generations of mothers whose own mothers said the same thing about

them. What her daughter considered empowering, Nasim considered exploitative—maybe not as exploitative as licking whipped cream off another girl, but humiliating nonetheless.

Shaida knew her mother's reservations. As they walked together back to Shaida's dorm after seeing *The Vagina Monologues*, under a star-studded night sky, Shaida left Nasim with these words: "I hope you know how proud I am of you. This could not have been easy for you to watch, but you really supported me."

The next night, she ran into Viktor at a hot-dog stand on campus and ignored him, even when he tried to make small talk with her. Her desire for revenge wasn't as strong as that of Nicole's, the GW sophomore. But Shaida left little doubt in Viktor's mind how angry at him she was.

Late in February, Shaida announced in her diary that she was happy and that, surprisingly, her good spirits had nothing to do with men. She had made friends with a group of international students whose backgrounds and interests resembled hers. They had visited the North Carolina Zoo in Asheboro one weekend, gone out for martinis one night, had long talks over dinner and were making plans for a trip to the Smoky Mountains in the spring.

And yet, she said, she missed flirting and hooking up. She watched her girlfriends, good-looking women, and saw how often men hit on them. After five months of celibacy, she wanted to get hit on, too, though not by just anybody. She hungered for a relationship of some sort even as she realized that she had become so abrasive in her feminism that few men would approach her.

When she first arrived at Duke, she had hooked up to test her appeal, different as she was from most other girls, and in her view, that had worked out okay. With Tomas she had taken a time-out from hooking up, and after Tomas, had resumed hooking up in search of the kind of intimacy she had had with him. When she didn't find it, she worried that she was becoming a "glorified fuckbuddy" to the guys she slept with, guys who cared for her slightly, perhaps, but never saw her as more than a sexy lay. She wanted to be more than that but couldn't figure out how to approach a guy in first gear rather than full throttle.

This can be one result of being in the habit of hooking up: You don't know how to do things differently once you realize you want more. Without a dating structure, you have had no experience in what an appropriate first step might be. And even if you ask a guy to go out for coffee, he may think you're hoping for more.

Shaida considered, on and off for several weeks, trying to start something with Clay, a senior in her new group. He was shy but friendly. Her friends told her he hadn't had sex for a year, so she was pretty sure he wouldn't make an unwanted move on her. The e-mail she sent me about him captured this generation's confusion:

"At first when we met, Clay and I clashed a lot. But now our fun arguing has become, I think, a kind of flirtation. Our mutual friends have commented on it to me. I trust Clay and I know for a fact he would never make a move on me."

The group would be going on a camping trip in a few weeks, she continued, so maybe something would happen there.

"I think what I feel with him is comfort and security and the possibility of great intimacy although he is nothing to me and I know for a fact that I'm nothing to him. I fear going after a guy so different from the men that I am used to. I mean, where do I even start?"

She never did figure out how to approach Clay, and he didn't pursue her. But a frat boy, Rob, entered the picture, briefly. Rob was a senior who came up to her late one weekend night at a club shortly before last call. She knew him casually, and when he kissed her, she kissed him back. They made out a little more and then he offered to give her a ride back to her dorm. When they arrived, she surprised herself by not inviting him back to her room. "It took all the self-control I had," she told me.

He used instant messaging to talk to her all the next week, then dropped by her room the next Friday and they made out—"completely sober," she noted. Her friends told her to invite him to an event, so she asked him to a jazz concert for the following Wednesday. He said he would arrive with his friends but never showed up. A few days later, he instant-messaged her to say his ex-girlfriend was coming into town and, in a roundabout way, asked Shaida to stay away from him until the ex left.

He tried to explain why. After he and his girlfriend first broke up, he had hooked up with someone else. "Then my ex came down to visit and the girl I'd hooked up with saw this, thought I was an asshole and found it necessary to tell my girlfriend that we had hooked up while I was in the bathroom at a bar . . . after which my ex punched me three times and left with one of my friends b/c she didn't want to leave with me, obviously."

He then told Shaida he'd like to see her after the ex left.

"I really don't want to be rebound," she responded.

"You're not rebound," he wrote.

"I just don't know how to read you," she responded.

"I'm a poker player . . . I don't give away my hand," he wrote.

Some years earlier, they might have been having this conversation in person and she could at least have read some clues from his face. But that night, she had to keep probing in brief lines of 12-point type.

At the end of their two-page IM session, Rob suggested that they try to meet up later in the week.

"Call me or IM me when you want to get together," she responded.

He never did, and to her surprise, she didn't care. Taking a line from a Pink Floyd song, she wrote in her diary that she had become "comfortably numb," though her description sounded anything but comfortable.

"It's unlike any kind of depression I have felt before," she wrote. "I don't sleep well; my eating pattern is different; I am constantly anxiety-filled and unfocused. I have gone from being oversexed and associating positive experiences with my vagina to being asexual and associating negative experiences."

Her diary was, I realized, her best friend. Unlike other girls I was following—Jamie at Duke and Nicole at GW, for example—she didn't have any really good girlfriends to "tend and befriend" her, as the anthropologists call it.

Without wise counsel from her peers or a mother like Sienna had, she continued to hook up. When a bluegrass band visited Durham, she came on to the drummer, who responded enthusiastically. "He likes feminists, is turned on by intellectual conversation and is a Marxist like me, which is weird because he looks like a pretty boy," she said. They were in a private home at the time, and went upstairs to a bedroom to make out. She told him she didn't want to have intercourse but he tried a couple of times anyway until she got really angry and he stopped.

"Why does this keep happening to me?" she wrote. "Did it happen to me in the past and I just didn't notice because I was too caught up in my dogma of sexual liberation? My biggest fear is that in the past I seemed strong enough and in control enough that guys didn't feel like they could violate me and get away with it. Now I'm unsure of myself. Is that what is giving men the idea that they can cross that line with me and that's okay? God, I miss the old Shaida."

Her social self-confidence was in decline just as she described it. One reason for the plunge, I learned as our year together drew to a close, went back to that first night I had accompanied her to Shooters.

Nathan had walked her to her car that night and told her that he wanted to hook up with her. She knew him slightly from the year before and found him mildly attractive so she said okay, but as they drove to her dorm, she warned him, "We are not going to have sex." She had had only one drink—a detail that would later become important—and was confident that she could enforce what she told him.

"Fine, I don't expect to," he replied.

Once in her room, they started taking off each other's clothes and making out, "all very normal for a hookup," she said. He took off her underwear and noticed that she wore a birth control patch. "That's stupid," he said. "You don't have a steady boyfriend to have sex with." He continued to razz her about different things, and she kept quiet until he started to penetrate her.

"Didn't I tell you we weren't going to have sex?" she asked.

In the hookup culture, some guys expect to be serviced.

"Can't I put it in for just a little bit?" he asked. "Only a few minutes, I swear."

She kept saying no, and under the law, he was obligated to stop. But he didn't.

"How can you write about sex and not have sex?" he asked.

The next time he penetrated her, she ripped open a condom package and handed over the contents. He put it on and continued what he was doing. She yelped in pain.

"I can't believe how sensitive you are! What's wrong with you?" he asked. She didn't feel strong enough to push him off, so she tried to enjoy it. But she couldn't.

"It hurts," she told him.

"Oh, I'm sorry," he said as he continued to thrust, adding, "I want to get you off."

"Good luck," she said. "I've never orgasmed before."

"What the fuck, you haven't orgasmed?" he gasped. "What's wrong with your body?"

His movements and coarse, ugly questions continued.

"Why aren't you enjoying this? Why aren't you moaning? You're a sex columnist!" Finally she was able to push him off and turn over on her stomach. He tried to cuddle up to her but she wouldn't let him.

The next morning she put on her bathrobe and said, "I'm going to class. You have to leave." Her thoughts were swirling. He had hurt her.

Or she had hurt herself by taking him to her room. Or they had both hurt each other and what do you call that?

What some might call it is rape. Nathan had penetrated her vagina despite the fact that she had clearly said "No."

Like most assault victims, she said nothing about the incident for a long time. Nine months after our visit to Shooters, she told her story publicly during a rally against sexual assault on the steps outside Duke Chapel. She did not name Nathan and left out some of the details, but she had already told enough people privately that her account eventually got back to Nathan. When students asked him about the incident, he denied he had assaulted her. She was so drunk at the time she couldn't possibly have remembered what happened, he said.

Her speech made quite an impression.

"You're the last person I would have expected to have this happen to," one young man said. She was the last person she would have expected in this situation, too, she told me, and that's why she had waited so long to explain what happened. She had always thought of herself as a conqueror, not a victim. "If I denied what happened, I wasn't one of those other, weaker girls," she said.

With the distance of almost a full school year, she could see that the persona she had adopted in college as a freshman and sophomore had almost destroyed her. Unlike Jamie in her first year at Duke, or Sienna and Anna in high school, she hadn't hooked up because that's what her friends were doing. She had hooked up—and made her sexual life a public affair—in an effort to force a debate on campus about the definition of power and who really possessed it. Several years later, the Duke campus would be forced to confront such questions in the wake of a major scandal involving its male lacrosse players and rape allegations brought by an exotic dancer the young men had hired for a private party. But when Shaida raised the same issues, few on campus were willing to listen or even engage her in constructive discussion.

Admittedly, her outspoken, sometimes abrasive, personality didn't inspire followers. At the same time, it's not at all clear that if it had, the women on Duke's campus would have rallied behind her. They were members of a generation who, in general, think individually rather than collectively. Donna Lisker, the Women's Center director, had been dealing with this fact for several years. As someone who had attended a women's college in the 1980s, she felt frustrated that Duke's young women didn't understand the power they could exert in their relationships with men if they worked together.

"If [sorority] Kappa Kappa Gamma told [fraternity] AEPi that they wouldn't come to an AEPi party unless the guys promised not to grope them, AEPi would stop groping women," she said. But sorority women, who set the standard for many nonsorority women, "are so invested in individual success that they can't see how to assert themselves as a group."

The idea of being a standard-bearer in several areas of campus life helped Shaida define who she was, but looking back on her first two years, she wondered if she should have confined herself to the safer issues of Middle Eastern politics and more general women's issues. She was learning the hard way that in order to inspire others to act in their own best interests, she had to do the same. Unfortunately, like many girls her age, she hadn't known at the time what was best for her. Shortly after our time together, she wrote:

The bra-burning feminist in me hates to admit this, but more often than not, after a hookup I woke up realizing that I didn't get what I wanted. Forget emotional satisfaction; the sex itself wasn't good. After a night of taking my sexuality and running with it, I didn't feel as sexually satisfied as I should have.

Sex isn't good unless it's intimate. Sex isn't good unless it means something. It doesn't necessarily need to mean "love" and it doesn't

necessarily need to happen in a relationship, but it does need to mean
intimacy and connection. . . . There exists a very fine line between
being sexually liberated and being sexually used.

But how were intimacy and connection different from lust? And how
could a woman experience either without knowing someone for a period
of time? These questions would pursue her in the years to come.

One thing she had learned—and it was significant—was that in crafting her own sexual persona, she did not want to adopt a male model of
hit-and-run. When sex is only about one person's enjoyment or need for
power, someone almost always gets hurt. And that someone is frequently
a woman who ends up blaming herself, particularly if she initiated the
action. The personal is not just political. It's also personal, sometimes too
much so. As some older feminists could have told her, sexual experimentation can be both fun and confidence-boosting, but only if the partners respect and trust each other and themselves.

"With Nathan I was anxious to be the person I had been, desired by
everyone," Shaida told me in one of our last meetings. "The first thing
I thought of as he entered me was, 'I need to get a condom,' when it
should have been 'I don't want to do this.' "

Parents and the Greenhouse Effect

CLEO'S STORY

"We've had everything handed to us."

—CLEO, TWENTY-ONE

No one in Cleo's circle of friends in Dallas ever thought she'd be the first to fall in love.

It wasn't that guys didn't try to hit on her. She was smart, fun and a real looker, with the black hair and dark eyes of her Greek heritage and a tall frame perfect for the fashionable dresses and three-inch heels she loved to wear. She always had plenty of guys around her; the problem was that the ones who wanted her, she wasn't interested in. And those she was interested in—one in high school in particular—didn't seem to want her.

"Everyone thought I'd be the drunken bridesmaid at all my friends' weddings," she told me at our first dinner.

Then along came Steven, a curly-haired young man of Irish-German descent whom she met her sophomore year at GW. They started dating in February of their junior year. He met her family; she spent Father's Day with his. The first time I had dinner with them, in the fall of their senior year, his blue-green eyes followed her every gesture. On that balmy September evening, sipping sangria at an outdoor Mexican café, they exuded the easy familiarity of a long-married couple.

"I love him so much," she said.

That worried her, though—a lot. Her mother, Daphne, was trying to arrange a job for her in Athens after graduation in the spring. She, on the other hand, had Paris and painting in mind. Whatever she did once school was over, she wasn't sure she wanted her plans to include Steven. "I don't want to lose the love of my life," she had told me privately, "but I also don't want to compromise my experiences for anybody."

Steven was ready for Europe or anywhere else that "Cles," as he called her, wanted to go. Eventually he dreamed of running for political office, but that could wait. He wasn't bothered by her independent spirit. "That's the best part about her," he said. But what if her independent plans didn't include him? "That would really suck," he told me that night. "I'm getting upset just thinking about it."

It wasn't the last time he'd suspect that their relationship was in jeopardy.

Cleo had told me almost three months earlier about her new relationship with Steven. She was the one who said, "It will suck if it's bad, but it will suck even more if it's good." Over the course of our year together, I came to understand what she meant—and the key, if unconscious, role her parents played in her ambivalence. As much as she tried to block them out, she couldn't help but hear, over and over, their messages about the perfect partner and the perfect time to become involved with him. Her parents, like others of their generation, had made a large financial and emotional investment in their daughter and didn't want her to make a mistake by attaching herself to the wrong guy. Like Shaida's mother, they preached the values of self-sufficiency and independence. Cleo didn't want to make a mistake, either, but she wanted a boyfriend. So she hung on to Steven, who, in her mind, was good enough. And she hooked up with other guys for two reasons: virtually everyone else she knew did, and Steven, as great as he was, wasn't Mr. Perfect. In her heart of hearts, she didn't want to just settle. She had never had to before.

SWING HARD

If there is a mantra that young women like Cleo have heard repeatedly from parents, teachers and each other, it is this: "Go for it. All of it." It is a theme of boundless opportunity sounded by the same feminists of the 1970s who, more than thirty years later, still place more value on professional success than on personal fulfillment. Cleo's mother wanted both for her daughters but emphasized the former. After law school, Daphne had accepted a job in a large law firm in Dallas and had practiced full-time ever since, even after giving birth to Cleo and, two years later, to Nicole. Daphne's paychecks paid for much of the house and pool, the private schools and her daughters' college education.

When she taped that quote to their desks—"How much you earn is determined by how much you learn"—she was preparing Cleo and Nicole to enjoy full lives with or without husbands. She sent them to all-girls' schools because she believed that single-sex education prepares girls to be leaders. She introduced her daughters to businesswomen and talked about the importance of networking. She was a relentless crusader. The year that Nicole was a freshman at GW and Cleo a junior, she sent them both the same clipping reviewing the work of top female CEOs. The year I was observing them, she mailed them copies of Virginia Woolf's *A Room of One's Own*.

One afternoon when Cleo was still in elementary school, Daphne passed by a baseball field and saw a boy taking batting practice while his grandfather pitched. "Swing hard," the grandfather advised. What a great idea, she thought, and she started using what would become one of her favorite expressions. No matter what you do in life, she told her daughters, "Swing hard."

Cleo's young life took on the shape and pace of her mother's. In addition to keeping an A average in high school, she played volleyball and rowed crew, held the position of "attorney" in the Mock Trial Club and edited the digital edition of the yearbook. At church, she played basketball on a state-championship team and was president of the youth group. Yet she was not sure, the entire year I followed her, that she wanted the same things from life that her mother wanted for her. "My mom has been amazing at her career," she said in one of our first interviews, "but I don't know what my work ethic is yet." In another interview she said, "I don't think I want the career or marriage my mom has."

She was very clear about what she was supposed to want. In this way, she was typical of a generation of young people who have had it drummed into them from the time they were toddlers that achievement in the outside world is the key to happiness. Achievement in one or two things will not do, however. Playing on the traveling lacrosse team or winning the young Tchaikovsky piano competition is not enough. The goal is to secure a place in a top college, then a top-ranked graduate school, then a lucrative profession. And given how many of you there are, they are told, the competition will be stiff. The more boxes you can check on any given application, the better your chances.

This generation of kids, or, more appropriately, their parents, might be characterized as "maximizers," a word first popularized in a *Scientific American* article. Maximizers must try everything and are rarely content, unlike "satisficers," an oddly spelled concept from that same essay, for whom most things are good enough. Not surprisingly, maximizers tend to live in families with at least a moderate amount of money.

National surveys have documented the accelerated lives of the young maximizers: They spend the equivalent of one more workday a week (7.5 hours) on homework than did children twenty years ago; two out of three take part in sports, extracurricular activities and volunteer work, usually all at one time; in high school, they cram music and other electives into lunch periods. Not surprisingly, given the pressure for girls to catch up with boys over the last two decades, young women spend more time than young men on these pursuits, with the exception of sports.

The stress-for-success that can result from these efforts has become so onerous that education officials in some parts of the country have started eliminating place markers such as class rank and capping the number of Advanced Placement courses one student can take. One honest principal in the Palo Alto, California, area, home of Stanford University, admitted the uphill battle facing her. "It's the nature of the community, the way people live their lives," she said.

I saw this ambition in high school students like Sienna, who had told her mother she would like to drop one of her sports but if she did, she wouldn't know what to do with herself. And I really saw it at universities such as GW and Duke, where the women swung hard, and not only in their classes. They'd spend spring break building houses with Habitat for Humanity and work twenty hours a week on campus, ringing up sales at the bookstore for books or beer money. On any night between seven and midnight, you could see them scattered across campus on their computers, e-mailing both a last-minute term paper and a chorus rehearsal schedule. They would IM three friends simultaneously about party plans, check their Facebook page and change their "away" message—all at the same time.

Not surprisingly, they extended their multitasking to their social lives. A Duke student-newspaper columnist wrote: "Taking on only one thing is an unchallenging and inefficient use of our time. What makes us really cool is that we apply this logic to social situations as well. . . . Why go to only one fraternity formal when you could go to one for each fraternity? Why hook up with just one [guy] when you could hook up with two?"

These young women expected to do a lot with their lives during and after college *and* do it very well. They were used to home runs; measly

grounders would not do. The examples their mothers had set both inspired and discouraged, and the supermoms didn't always wear business suits.

I remember standing in the kitchen with Sienna's mother, Beth, as she
was preparing for a few of Sienna's friends to come over before the
homecoming dance. Standing in her spotless kitchen, preparing seltzer
water in tall wineglasses and slicing a lime, she admitted that as a full-time
homemaker, she worked hard to keep everything "in the range of perfect." As she spoke, she pulled already glistening sterling silver ice tongs
out of a drawer and reached under the sink to get the silver polish.

Parents are not the only culprits; perfectionism in this country is a
viral infection nourished by the Madison Avenue–inspired notion that we
can eliminate facial wrinkles and sexual dysfunction. Alicia, a junior at
Duke, spoke to me about this. She had been adopted as a baby from
Korea by a couple in a middle-income community outside Washington,
D.C. Her parents wanted her to do well in school but didn't push her to
excel to the extent that Cleo's parents pushed Cleo. Nonetheless, as her
high school career drew to a close, she was pulling down a near-perfect
GPA, playing three sports, including competitive gymnastics, and teaching Sunday school. She was named valedictorian—and she had a nervous breakdown.

She started seeing a psychologist, who helped her enormously, and
she enrolled in Duke, a campus full of students as ambitious as she. It
wasn't until she took a course in leadership as a junior that she started to
understand fully how she had been affected by such a driven culture.

In a paper for that course, she wrote:

Over the years I have pointed many fingers to try and explain my
desperate need to be perfect. I thought of gymnastics, the sport to
which I devoted fourteen years of my life, and wondered if the constant training to achieve the perfect body and the elusive 10 had

somehow taken over my brain. I thought of my parents, and how they had pushed me to abide by strict religious values they hold dear (on pain of going to hell).

She concluded in the paper that "no one was asking me to be perfect; I was demanding perfection of myself." Privately, however, she told me she knew that she hadn't gotten to that point completely on her own. "If people are telling girls to be smart or beautiful or accomplished, we will find a way to be all those things."

The task force at Duke that looked at the status of women on campus reported the same thing. Undergraduates told committee members that their campus environment was characterized by "effortless perfection": the expectation that girls would be "smart, accomplished, fit, beautiful and popular, and that all of this would happen without visible effort."

With all they do or feel they should be doing, how can we possibly expect girls like Alicia or Cleo to find the time and energy to pursue a romantic interest successfully? It's not at all clear. Listen to Alicia again:

> Dating is a drain on energy and intellect, and we are overworked, overprogrammed and overcommitted just trying to get into grad school, let alone getting married. It's rare to find someone who would, from the perspective of being single and not in a serious relationship, want to put their relationships over their academics/future. I don't even know that relationships are seen as an integrated part of this whole "future" idea. Sometimes I think they are on their own track that runs parallel and that we feel can be pushed aside or drawn closer at our whim.

When Alicia's and Cleo's mothers were the age of their daughters, college was about finding your life's work *and* someone to marry. Virtually everyone, guys as well as girls, followed the same timetable. For Alicia, Cleo and their classmates, the search for a marriage partner comes after the partying has wound down, the career is under way and the college loans are paid off. It's not difficult to see why, for some, life is a Jane Austen novel: over when you get married.

Sigmund Freud is said to have believed that a happy life is made up of two things: love and work. Society has asked these young women to choose between the two, and they've chosen work, at least for the short term. Large majorities say they want to be married, but if current trends hold, they'll be in their late twenties or early thirties before they marry, and most will continue to work at least part-time.

Cleo expanded upon her mother's notion of why work is important. It's not just because drawing a paycheck will make her independent, she said. Working also will help make her a perfect partner. "How can you be your husband's intellectual equal if you don't work?" she asked. Long gone are the days that Jane Austen wrote about, when the right husband, carefully chosen, would correct a woman's flaws. We salute their passing, but should spend more time figuring out how to help girls be satisfied with something short of perfection. Perhaps we start by saying a B on a test isn't the end of the world, being a size 8 instead of a 4 is fine— and dating a guy for a while (or "hanging out," if that's preferred) can be loads of fun. He doesn't have to be perfect, and neither does the relationship.

Unlike her younger sister, Nicole, Cleo was always a soft touch. She was the one who stood back in preschool and let bigger girls muscle ahead of her in the water-fountain line, unlike Nicole, who sent them running. She was the one who, when her third-grade girlfriend had to get her long hair cut off against her will, begged Daphne to cut her locks so that her playmate might feel better. Where Nicole snapped black-and-white photographs as a hobby in high school, Cleo stroked canvas in richly colored oils.

As big a heart as she had, she had had several romantic crushes in high school and was still thinking about a couple of those boys. Jack was one of them. He was a hunk in her opinion and in the opinion of the girls she ran with. Blond-haired, green-eyed and athletic, he had an air of studied aloofness broken occasionally by a half-smile. He didn't date in high school, as far as Cleo or her friends knew, and as a high school senior, Cleo decided to see if she could spur his interest. On a late summer day, right before the gang split up to enroll in different universities, they gathered at Cleo's house for a pool party. Cleo bet her girlfriends that she could crack Jack that night, and she did, showing him into the bathroom at three in the morning and making out, though not going all the way.

Jack departed for Harvard, Cleo for GW, and they flirted by e-mail freshman year. They decided to spend the coming summer together as camp counselors in Texas and made a list of all the things they'd do: take a road trip to the beach, watch Disney movies, ride his motorcycle. Once they arrived at camp, the young campers teased them about being boyfriend and girlfriend and neither denied it, but as the summer wore down, Jack began pulling away. During the last week, Cleo told Jack that she loved him—the first time she had said that to any guy—and received a barely audible grunt in return. She returned to GW disappointed and angry. She had fantasized about having a real relationship with Jack but realized that wasn't going to happen any time soon. Her dream for the perfect romance dashed, she gave her virginity away to a visiting student from a college in North Carolina whom she didn't like that much.

"It was a typical first time," she said. "Horrible."

She met Steven that year through Steven's friend John, with whom she hooked up, on and off, for several months. When she learned that John was seeing another girl, she cut him off. She flirted with Steven, but he was attached to a girl in his hometown. He stayed attached until the spring of their junior year when, one evening in the kitchen of an off-campus house, Cleo put her hands on his shoulders and said, "I really want to kiss you." That was that. They spent the summer apart, then picked back up in the fall of senior year.

In October of that year, Cleo flew to Boston to see old friends, including Jack. She ended up sharing an ice cream cone with him and talking for more than an hour. One of Jack's friends who was with them at the time commented afterward to her about the "chemistry" that she and Jack seemed to share. She knew it was true. He was like a magnet, pulling her toward him whenever they were in the same room. He obviously felt something for her as well but couldn't express what it was.

Back at school, she and Steven resumed their relationship. He was an attentive lover and pleased her more in bed than anyone else ever had. She never felt she could fulfill his desires in the way that she would have liked, but he said he was satisfied. Steven's best friend started telling people that Cleo and Steven were going to get married. This freaked Cleo out, and it really freaked out her mother.

Daphne and Niko, Cleo's father, met Steven for the first time in the early fall of Cleo's senior year. The two families dined together at a restaurant on the Georgetown waterfront, and Daphne told Cleo afterward that Steven seemed like a good person. "But," she warned, "you two are getting too serious. You've got plans after graduation." Daphne didn't approve of Jack, either, and questioned why Jack had never had a real girlfriend. Cleo had heard these warnings about guys from her mother for years. "Maybe it's her way of protecting me," Cleo told me, "but it's incredibly annoying."

Annoying, perhaps, but it also enabled Cleo to justify seeing guys other than Steven by saying, "I'm not ready to be serious." According to various surveys, between one-third and one-half of college students say they've cheated while in a relationship. But what is cheating in the unhooked culture? It was unclear what Cleo thought it was. A kiss? No.

Fondling? No. Oral sex? Not sure. Whatever it was, it did not escape her attention that she was acting the part of the rogue while Steven had assumed the role of faithful wife. "He does whatever I want," she told me. "I'm ashamed to say I have used that fact sometimes."

One day in midfall, she tried to break up with him, saying, "I don't have time to balance everything." He convinced her to come back, saying, "I'm sorry you are stressed. If you are sad, it's like I'm living that same pain." She couldn't stand to see him hurt, and she had to admit that it was nice to have someone who loved her unconditionally—with no parentlike expectations that she be perfect. So she continued to date Steven, e-mail Jack and every once in a while, when out with her girlfriends at a bar, sneak a kiss or two with a good-looking stranger. It was a pattern that was hard to abandon.

I began to understand Cleo's feelings for Steven after I listened to her mother describe her own youthful relationships. In college, Daphne had believed, like so many of her contemporaries, that sex, freely expressed, was a symbol of power for women as well as men. Unlike her daughters, she and her pals at college didn't worry about HIV or other serious infections. "We could go to Planned Parenthood and get the pill. Whoever smiled at you in class was a candidate. I did not have serious boyfriends. I always had Niko in the back of my mind, but I did not deprive myself of the companionship."

Companionship. That's what Cleo and Steven shared, a deep, intimate and powerful companionship. But where was the all-consuming passion that Cleo felt for Jack? Steven felt it for her, that was clear. Why didn't she feel it for him? And what did it mean for them in the long run? These were questions Cleo discussed regularly with her best friend, Jess. But she didn't really talk about them with her mom because she knew how cautiously her mother approached the subject of love.

Who doesn't remember her or his first real romantic crushes? "Ah, the quality of them. They influenced who I became," recalled Lloyd Kolbe, a health education professor at the University of Indiana in his fifties. I was interviewing him in a small classroom during a break at a conference on adolescent health. His face lit up at the question like a fifteen-year-old boy's. "I still have dreams about them."

Kolbe, formerly an adolescent health director at the Centers for Disease Control and Prevention, noted that most older adults, parents included, would rather talk about almost anything other than their early loves. Even sex, as awkward a topic as it is, comes up more often in conversations, he said. "We demean first love, deny it, trivialize it, and so our young people trivialize it. We lose our opportunity to talk about real things, like the difference between lust and love. Sex is part of it, but not the central part of it."

My sense is that as their daughters get older, parents begin worrying that crushes may become *too* significant, distracting girls from more important things like algebra homework. The physical risks of sex can be addressed with a pill, patch and condom, but there's no contraception available for the heart. So they signal their girls, either consciously or unconsciously, to "love moderately," as Daphne put it, lest that college scholarship go to someone else.

Several years ago, social commentator Kay Hymowitz suggested, in an essay titled "The L Word: Love as Taboo," that Americans' "profoundly rationalistic vision of human relations" was partly the product of feminism, "which feared that love and equality were incompatible." She quoted Marilyn French's *The Women's Room*, a best-selling novel in 1977 in which a character called love "a lie to keep women happy in the kitchen so they won't be asked to do what men are always doing." She also noted that feminist antipathy toward love surfaced as early as the mid-nineteenth century and traveled into the twentieth century on the shoulders of college-educated women and men who replaced passion and its more negative sidelines like jealousy with "shared interests, common background and sexual pleasure."

As I re-read Hymowitz's essay, I realized that several of the young women I was observing labored under French's impression that they couldn't love deeply and passionately and live the independent, meaningful lives their parents told them they wanted and that many of them did, in fact, desire. Dating couples rarely said "I love you." They might be engaging in oral sex but wouldn't think of holding hands as they walked across campus. They were having sex but not making love.

Perhaps Cleo couldn't give herself completely to Steven because he wanted to go into politics and she didn't want to be a politician's wife. But it appeared to be more than that. The rational side of her loved Steven; the irrational side lusted after Jack. She wasn't sure she could find the qualities of both in a third person—or what she'd do if she did. Sometimes she wanted to confess everything to Steven. Because she didn't, she worried that he would find out about Jack in some other way, and she knew the damage to him then would be far worse. One thing was very clear: No one other than her friends was helping her sort through her feelings or navigate this treacherous landscape. She was a spontaneously loving, deeply caring—and very confused—young woman.

Cleo had no vision of what good love, good sex and meaningful work looked like in combination. Like so many parents, hers refrained from demonstrating affection for each other in front of their children, leaving Cleo and Nicole to view marriage as, at best, a manageable service contract.

Parents can be reluctant to open a full two-way dialogue about love, lest they have to admit their own indiscretions and marital disappointments. They want to appear in control and be able to offer solutions even as their kids become adults. They do what they feel comfortable doing: help a maturing child devise a budget, furnish an apartment, maybe find a first job. Giving advice about emotional intimacy is some-

thing else, particularly if their own experiences have been less than perfect. As a result, kids grow up depending on parents for help with everything except what may be life's most fundamental need: to love and be
loved by a life partner.

Daphne, in fact, was more forthright than many mothers are. "Love
is not forever," she told her daughters. "I've had disappointments with
your father. Absolutely nothing is guaranteed."

Young women from divorced or single-parent homes may have even
less to go on. The AARP in 2003 surveyed divorced and single Americans forty and older about the quality of their love—and sex—lives.
The responses were not encouraging. Those polled said they were in
search of companionship, not commitment (what an AARP magazine editor called "deep like" rather than love). They valued their freedom. And
they were lonely, the women more so than the men. Sixty percent of the
women in their fifties said they had not had sex, been touched, been embraced or felt loved once in the past six months. Surely they wouldn't
want to admit that to their children. Just as surely, they wouldn't want
that to happen to their children later in middle age.

Of course, past generations of parents weren't exactly candid about
love or sex, either. But there were generally accepted rules back then
about what to do and not do sexually. These standards restricted young
women more than young men, by no means a fair deal, but they at least
allowed women time and space to consider what kind of partners they
wanted to love and what that love should look like. The guardrails have
vanished, except among certain religious communities, and in their place
is an increasingly sophisticated marketing industry pushing sex-toy workshops and T-shirts that read "Juicy" and "Cunning Linguist."

The consequence is this: Because kids hear and participate in so few
adult discussions about love, and rarely see examples of love among the
adults they know, they come to believe that the sex they see around them
is love. And when they find out that it isn't, they can only resort to con-

versations with each other or glib self-help books like *He's Just Not That into You* and *Be Honest—You're Not That into Him Either.*

It occurred to Cleo, as she watched the evolution of her sister Nicole's relationship with Michael and her mother's increasingly positive reaction to it, that Daphne might be more concerned about Cleo's choice of men than about the idea of commitment itself. Cleo said her mom had a complex series of goals and objectives for her daughters, and one of them was that they marry Greeks, preferably wealthy Greeks. A medical student or lawyer would be nice. Neither Steven nor Jack fit her bill of particulars.

Could it be that parents unconsciously endorse hooking up as a stop-gap measure until the partner of their child's dreams—or perhaps more honestly, their dreams for their child—comes along?

THE GREENHOUSE EFFECT

Something seemed odd as I pulled up in front of Cleo's home for the first time. I realized with a start that on this broad, flat Dallas street, bordered by immaculate green lawns and tall, graceful oak trees, mine was the only car. Not another human being could be seen.

It turned out that homeowners parked their cars behind their homes and normally entered their houses through the back doors. Family and community life took place indoors and on backyard patios. "My girls were never allowed to play in the front yard," Daphne told me.

They also were never allowed to walk to school, and were driven to piano lessons, Greek school and all their other extracurricular activities. When they wanted to ride bikes, their parents rode bikes with them.

Cleo and Nicole never thought of themselves as confined because every other child they knew lived the same way. Daphne rationalized the limits she placed on the girls as necessary for their safety. But occasionally she felt a twinge of regret at how different their growing up was from her own.

During the 1950s and early 1960s, her father went to work every day at his advertising business in a small Texas town and her mom stayed in their split-level home with her and her younger sister. When she wasn't in school, she was outside roller-skating or riding her bike all over town until dark. She had chores to do at home and strict limits on how quickly she could grow up. Shaving her legs at twelve, for example, was out of the question, although eventually her mother gave in.

Cleo and Nicole's childhood was much different, and not just in their daily comings and goings. As Daphne was the main breadwinner, she left for work every morning just as the kids were getting up. Their dad was frequently the one to pick them up after school, although Daphne managed to do that occasionally. When Cleo was about six months old, Daphne hired a nanny who lived with them for five years.

They attended exclusive schools and ran around in packs of girls and boys from other exclusive schools. They and their friends had frequent parties. As they grew older and their taste in clothes turned to Burberry and Nicole Miller, Daphne would slip them her credit card to go shopping at Saks or Neiman Marcus. She wanted them to learn the value of restraint, but she didn't want them to look or feel too out of step with their friends, many of whom came from wealthier families.

Cleo summed up her parents' generosity this way: "We've had everything handed to us."

Indeed, many in their generation have. They are spectacular specimens raised in glass houses that are temperature-controlled and as disease-free as humanly possible. It is a natural desire of most parents to protect their children, and these children have been protected as no generation before them by parents who can afford it. When young they are bathed in antibacterial soap and showered with educational toys. When they go to school and appear to be failing a course, their teacher may be asked to reevaluate his or her grading policy. If their mind wanders, they're taken to doctors who prescribe Adderall, and if they have trouble sitting still, Ritalin. Schools lay cushioned rubber on outdoor play-grounds so kids won't skin their knees when they fall and remove soda and snack machines because too many are getting obese. Principals cancel classes at the first threat of snow because they fear parents would sue if there was an accident on the way to school, and of course if the buses can't run, kids would—God forbid—have to find some other way to get to school.

Their opportunities for learning how to be responsible for their own wants are few. As teenagers, they get allowances ranging from twenty-five dollars a week to one hundred dollars a week to be spent largely at their discretion. Some take jobs in high school to buy the CDs they covet, but others don't (Cleo and Nicole didn't), their parents' philosophy being that their classes, school projects and after-school activities *are* their work.

They are, in short, the heroines of their parents' lives before they ever get to college, and once in college, they have no reason to believe that will change. The results are encouraging on some fronts. According to those who study generational differences, these young women (and young men) are, as a whole, optimistic rule-followers who value school and trust authority figures. They may make good employees. But will they make good lovers or good marriage partners? They have learned little about taking risks, making tough choices, attending to others' needs or weathering disappointment on their own—in short, some of the tools they will need to forge strong, intimate bonds and forgo connections that are not good for them.

For girls whose mothers have decided to make raising their children their profession, the attention can be particularly intense. Jamie, the Duke senior, talked about this a good bit. Her mother made elaborate dinners for her and her brother almost every night as they were growing up. If Jamie wanted a certain dress for a dance or a certain piece of furniture for her room, her mom spent days searching discount retailers and online shopping sites. This attention continued through Jamie's college career.

Jamie wasn't complaining as she told me these stories. She had friends, she said, whose mothers did even more for them, including one whose mother composed her résumé and filled out her job applications. When baby-boomer parents first started reading to this generation, one of the books they read was Marlo Thomas's *Free to Be You and Me*, a story/songbook celebrating diversity. A more appropriate title might have been *Free to Be Me, Thanks to You*.

Adolescence has always been about crafting one's singular identity, and until twenty or so years ago, it was assumed that as adolescents got older, they did most of the crafting. They would, with only limited assistance, finish school, get a full-time job, marry, start a family and become adults in the eyes of the world—and, more important, in their own eyes. This would all happen somewhere between eighteen and twenty-four.

Today it's more like thirty or thirty-four—prolonged adolescence, researchers call it, or emerging adulthood. Many young people either go to graduate school after college or move back in with their parents. Some do get apartments on their own but still receive financial assistance from Mom and Dad. There are some sound reasons for parental assistance— high prices of housing and health insurance among them. But is this overall a good development? Do young people need to be able to take that much time to experiment in their search for what—and who—will make them happy? Are they not growing up because they don't know how? Or because parents and the rest of adult society won't let them?

Theirs is a highly individualistic—for some, even self-centered— ethic that has been magnified by another gift of the older generation: the computer chip. Parents know that their children cannot compete in school without a computer at home. Soon, the single-family computer morphs into a computer in every bedroom, along with one or more video-game players, DVD players, a CD burner, an iPod and not just a cell phone but a cell phone that takes pictures, sends and receives e-mails and transmits instant messages. With the help of these new best friends, young people can craft a world exactly to their liking, outside the purview of their parents—a novel experience indeed.

One can't help but think that the lifelong focus on them helps explain why the unhooked culture thrives. Writing in *The Harvard Crimson* about cheating on tests and in relationships, a student said: "At Harvard, we know competition and many of us know how to prioritize ourselves—our needs—above all. . . . Some people are drawn to these behavioral patterns more than others. It's those who are imbued with a high sense of personal value. You see the world as your oyster, and you think there is nothing wrong with taking everything that world has to offer."

INDECISION

By the middle of her senior year, Cleo had a 3.76 grade point average, her best ever at GW. She was studying for the foreign service exam that her father insisted she take even though she wasn't at all sure she wanted to be a diplomat. She also was anticipating her one-year anniversary with Steven. He wouldn't tell her where he was taking her to dinner but promised it would be special. And it was. First, they dined at an expensive Middle Eastern restaurant and killed off an expensive bottle of pinot noir. Then they went to a café for carrot cake and more drinks and, after that, to a Japanese bar. Steven spent about two hundred dollars that night, so much that on Valentine's Day, he had no money and they had to stay at his house and watch a movie.

Through all of this, her conscience bothered her—not, for the moment, because of anything she had done, but because she was thinking about Jack at least as much as about Steven. How was it possible to have strong feelings about two people at the same time?

Over Christmas, Steven had flown to Dallas to visit for four days. He had never been to the South, and she enjoyed showing him around the Dallas–Fort Worth area. Steven watched her carefully as they went out with her old friends, including Jack. After Steven left, she had coffee with another old friend, Trent, who confided that he liked her. Cleo told this to Steven once they were both back at school. Steven's response was not what she was expecting.

"You know who really still has feelings for you?" he asked. "Jack."

"I wanted to say, 'Oh really? What did he look like that makes you say that?' But I didn't," she told me later.

Cleo and Jack had hung out together after Steven flew home to Pennsylvania. Jack had told Cleo that he had dated a couple of girls at Harvard but that the relationships didn't last long or mean anything. He also had said he wanted to take a trip to Washington as a tourist, and she offered to let him stay in her dorm suite.

Cleo admitted to me that she didn't know whether she really liked Jack, or just the idea of chasing him. She didn't exercise the same control over him that she did with Steven, and that both annoyed and intrigued her. I saw her ambivalence differently. It seemed to me that Jack was Cleo's first choice and that, if he were available, she would drop Steven in a heartbeat. But Jack wasn't completely there for her, and because Steven was, and presented a more-than-acceptable second choice, she was trying to keep her options open. It was as if she had found a Porsche she really loved but could take it out only for an occasional joyride, so she didn't want to dump the cute and serviceable Beetle.

What she was seeking was some sort of intellectual construct that would tell her that was okay.

Shortly after she returned to campus in January, she and I met at a Starbucks for lunch. She was as anxious as I had ever seen her. Her course load leading up to graduation was heavy: European history, French literature, political science methods, graduate-level economics and the global development of public health. But that wasn't what was eating at her. This was: When Jack came to visit, she wanted to ask him straight out if he liked her as more than a friend.

"What if he said no?" I asked her.

"What if he said yes?" she answered, sounding more like an uncertain seventh-grader than a young woman about to graduate from college.

Once asked, the question would force her to confront issues of trust and betrayal with both boys. If Jack indicated strong feelings for her, she would have to tell Steven, who would be devastated. But Jack would know she had cheated on Steven to be with him and would have cause to wonder whether she would cheat on him. Trying to bring some form to her thoughts, she sketched out briefly—whether for my sake or hers, it wasn't clear—several differences between the two.

Steven came from a loving, two-parent home. He was comfortable with himself and "out to please people, to make them feel comfortable and loved." Jack's mom and dad divorced when Jack was five. Jack grew up with his mom, whom he loved a lot, but he didn't see much of his dad and was disappointed by him over the years. "That's why he doesn't trust people or himself," she said. "Jack does what he feels comfortable doing. He's not selfish; he's just confused. He has had to change a lot more than Steven in college." Ah, a slight variation on the old story, I thought to myself: My guy may be a jerk, but he's *my* jerk, and I can change him. Jack wasn't a jerk, but he also didn't appear to be exactly who Cleo thought he was or wanted him to be.

Steven, on the other hand, was exactly as he appeared. She said he had asked her to remain his girlfriend through the end of the year and that she had agreed. "I don't want to ruin his last semester."

Jack postponed his visit to Washington, and by early April, three months after our conversation at Starbucks, it appeared that Cleo's feelings for Steven were changing once again and that the two of them were getting closer. They had visited the Yucatán Peninsula, in Mexico, over spring break with friends from GW and enjoyed each other's company. "We're at such a good point in our relationship, more like best friends," she told me. "We understand each other really well. We know where each other is at any given point in the day. I'll make him breakfast before class, or write him little notes if I'm going to pull an all-nighter. At first I was not okay with the fact that I have a boyfriend. Now I'm more than okay with that."

Typically, as graduation approaches, college seniors begin making a list of coeds they've had their eye on but never actually seduced. In that circus atmosphere, and given her "maximizing" tendencies, it was unlikely that Cleo was going to stay faithful to Steven in the last couple of months of college. And she didn't, in the strictest sense of the word.

One night after spring break, she and her girlfriends went to a bar and she ran into a guy she'd had a crush on in the past. She kissed him for a while before deciding, "Ooh, I don't want that." The next week Jack e-mailed her to say he was coming to visit near the end of April.

Before he arrived, a young track star from Greece, Ari, whom she had met at camp several years earlier, swung through D.C. to see her. He had brought two guys with him, and their little group stopped by Steven's house for a while before going out to the clubs. Steven didn't accompany them, and Ari and Cleo ended up closing down the bar at two-thirty in the morning and returning to her dorm room where they slept in her bed. They kissed and talked about how they liked each other, concluding that their plans after graduation prevented anything serious from developing.

"I'm really glad I got to see Ari," she wrote in an e-mail, "but my thoughts always float back to Jack at the end. It's still the idea of Jack that's most appealing out of everyone, even my boyfriend and even probably the best-looking GREEK guy I have ever kissed in my life. So I'm definitely excited by his visit and the chance to get this over with! We've been e-mailing each other back and forth this past week. . . . He said that he visited Kansas City to see his dad and that one area 'really reminded

him of me,' and that he was 'pumped to come to D.C.,' whatever
that means."

Cleo's frenzied running between Steven and other boys reminded me
of something Jamie had said when Austin was pulling away from her.
"I've never been in a situation where I didn't know the right thing to do."
Cleo was precisely at the same point, although in her case she was the one
pulling away. Some girls don't know how to start a relationship; Cleo
didn't know how to end one. The unhooked culture gives little guidance
on either.

As she saw it, she didn't need to make any firm decisions. Marriage
was far in the future, so why did Steven need to be so serious? He might
be the perfect partner—despite what her mother thought—but how
would she know without trying other boys?

She also was feeling that Steven didn't really listen to or try to understand her reservations. She had secured the promise of a full-time job
in community health in nearby Alexandria, Virginia, after graduation,
and this gave her the confidence to break up with Steven again a few days
before Jack was to visit, although it was unclear, as relationships often
are with this generation, how long the break would last. "I have to do this
because Steven wouldn't do it himself," she told me.

Jack arrived for a two-day visit and they walked all over Washington, visiting the National Cathedral, the gardens near the White House
and other sights that he had never seen. At Christmas, she had told
him that she loved Steven but didn't know if she was *in* love with him.
This time, she said that she and Steven were on a break. Both things
were true and, she hoped, made her appear less desperately in love
with Jack. She and Jack slept in the same bed in her dorm room on the
nights he was in town. He was about to take a job in Chicago, and they
talked about her flying out there to see him sometime over the coming
summer. They made out but didn't go all the way, and in her mind, that
prevented her from being simply the dreaded "friend with benefits"—

a label that usually foreclosed anything more serious from developing. Making out, in her mind and in the minds of her friends, appeared to mean not much more than shaking hands.

Cleo introduced me to Jack late on a Saturday morning during a break in their sightseeing. She took off for a while, leaving me to talk with the guy who had consumed so much of her thinking. Jack, wearing khaki shorts and a bright orange University of Texas T-shirt that Cleo had given him, was both friendly and guarded. He admired Cleo, that much was clear. "She's very pretty, fun, easy to talk to," he said, "and that's important 'cause I'm a shy guy." He continued, without prompting, "She's smart, a good conversationalist, and can make fun of herself. When some people make a mistake, they get flustered. She just laughs it off. That's important to me, too.

"She doesn't play games with me. When we were dating, if something was on her mind, she'd say it."

I took note of the word "were." Clearly, in his mind they weren't dating, which left me thinking that to him, dating meant more than seeing the sights of Washington together or even hooking up. He told me he had had three "girlfriends" in college, each for about a month, but that they weren't "worth dating." Apparently, to Jack, "dating" was a lot like being engaged to be married. He later talked about two good male friends who had been in relationships with the same girls since freshman year. His view of this? "They've wasted four years."

"To find someone, that's really scary," he said. "Everyone wants that, but it's for the rest of your life." Here it was again, from a young man this time, the view that either you hooked up or you were "married." There was nothing in between.

The morning after our conversation, he flew back to Boston without committing to anything. Cleo was left wondering again how much he liked her, but she said she wasn't too upset. By now she was used to his indecisiveness.

The following Thursday, the day before Cleo and I were to fly to Dallas to celebrate Easter at her home, Steven showed up at her dorm pleading with her to reconsider her decision to break up. "I'm so desperately in love with you, I can't walk away," he said.

She described the scene for me as our plane headed south. "I so wish I could say the same thing," she said. "But I want to have a chance to date Jack again. This time is for me!"

A week after she returned from Dallas, she gave Steven one last chance. They spent the last three weeks of school together, studying for finals, finishing papers, partying and finding an apartment for her. One evening shortly after graduation, I arrived at the new apartment to pick them up for dinner. They were both moving a little sluggishly, which they explained by saying that the night before, they and a couple dozen of their friends had gathered at Steven's house and played hours of "Capture the Case," a college version of "Capture the Flag" involving cases of Bud Light instead of a flag. The crowd had consumed more than ten cases of beer, 240 cans. Letting go of childhood, like letting go of childhood partners, was harder than they had imagined it would be.

When I was Cleo's age, I was working in television, preparing to go to graduate school in journalism and dating a guy who would become my husband. I felt very much like an adult and never questioned that I could do it all. Cleo and others her age didn't seem to have that same confidence. I came across a column from the Duke *Chronicle* the night I had dinner with Cleo and Steven that expressed well the uncertainty I had observed in Cleo and other young women. It was written by a junior, Anne Katharine Wales, who said, in part:

> At Duke, we're on a fast-paced track, taking 200-level classes, getting internships with big companies and making connections with the people who are shaping the world in ways we admire. Our dreams are becoming a reality.

This is what we've always wanted.

But during college we're also meeting people who open our eyes to new ideas, who show us the world in an amazing way. . . . Somewhere along the line most of us have gotten really close to someone, maybe even fallen in love. . . . For some reason, this scares us beyond belief. Somehow this doesn't fit with our plan of achieving our dreams. We want to be independent; we want to go off and change the world in our own way. But we never planned on falling for someone else. When we graduate as seniors, most people who are dating are faced with the question of either marrying or breaking up because one person is going to graduate school in California while the other is working in New York. . . .

Society tells us to follow our dreams, our University tells us that success is working at that job we've always wanted, and our parents tell us to do whatever our heart desires (although they secretly hope their $40,000 a year in tuition doesn't go to waste). We have career counselors telling us how to get that internship, get accepted to med school and get that high-paying job. But no one is telling us how to work our feelings into this equation for success.

Sometimes I wish I were five again, when I was afraid of monsters living in my closet, my only job was to run outside and play and the only decisions I had to make involved what kind of ice cream I wanted for dessert.

My last meeting with Cleo and Steven together, like our first one, took place at an outdoor café, this time a French one. As we sat there waiting for salade niçoise and crêpes, Steven said he didn't mind talking about Cleo's weekend with Jack. He didn't know exactly what happened between them and didn't really want to know. If Jack had come to visit Cleo two years earlier and if she had wanted to take a break then, that would have been it for him, he said. But he was older now, and he had decided

with a start one morning, high on several cups of coffee, that Cleo was
not playing him but really having second thoughts.

"I might have felt better for a day had I told her off," he said that
night, "but she is the one who makes me feel better every day."

They explained their plans. Steven was moving to Philadelphia the
next day to volunteer in a local political campaign. Cleo was staying in
Washington. Their connection would be what their generation calls an
"open relationship," meaning that they were free to hook up with other
people but would also see each other from time to time and be what
Steven called "brutally honest" about their feelings for their relationship.

"We have to figure out if this relationship was just good for college
or something we want to go back to in a couple of years," Cleo explained.

They knew that the social scene they were about to enter after college was just as formless as the one they were leaving and would make
answering their question difficult. This bothered them both.

"Hooking up affects us because people don't take our relationship
seriously," Steven said.

Cleo nodded. "If a guy hits on me and I say I have a boyfriend, he'll
say, 'So?' And if he's hot, some of my girlfriends say, 'Go for it!' "

They were sitting across from each other at a small forest-green metal
table, oblivious to the waiter who was to serve our food. Within twenty-
four hours, Steven would be on a train and Cleo would be on her own
for the first time in her life.

"I know I have to do this," she said in a near whisper. "You're supposed to find yourself, be alone after college." Her eyes watered, much
as Steven's eyes had almost a year before when he thought about Cleo
going to Europe without him.

Steven touched her knee. "What would you like to eat, Cles?"

The College Environment

VICTORIA'S STORY

"If I start 'talking to' someone, he's not going to wait
two months to make out. It's really hard to find someone
to be patient and who respects you that much."

—VICTORIA, EIGHTEEN

The two girls slipped into the freshman women's orientation session at Duke side by side and sat as close together as their folding chairs would allow. Jocelyn was a comely, light-brown-skinned girl with gorgeous black hair that spiraled over her shoulders. She looked twenty, maybe twenty-one. Her companion, Victoria, was petite, with golden skin, a baby face and braids that made her appear not a day over fourteen.

They had come to hear Shaida and other upperclasswomen describe what kind of social life they could expect on campus. The advice-givers had a lot to say, much of it contradictory. "If you go out, ask a guy friend to watch out for you" was one, followed shortly thereafter by "Guys are predators." "If you want to hook up, that's great, but if you want it because you're interested in the guy, watch out" was another. This was followed by "We're going to talk about monogamy even though it might seem strange." At that last statement, Victoria gave her friend a questioning look.

Monogamy was all Victoria knew. She came from Johnson City, Tennessee, a community of 55,000 in the foothills of the Smoky Mountains. Her father, Albert, a Haitian refugee, was a physician specializing in internal medicine. Her mother, Marie, also from Haiti, had made a gracious home for Victoria and Victoria's sister and brother. Her cooking was famous among Victoria's friends, and one of the most eager of diners during Victoria's senior year in high school was Victoria's boyfriend, Nicholas.

Photos of Nicholas covered the white walls of Victoria's dorm room when I first met her. She told me she slept in one of his shirts, which smelled faintly of his cologne. When she made her bed every morning, the last thing she did was place a stuffed Daisy Duck on her pillow, a gift he brought her from Disney World.

She and Nicholas had parted after high school graduation, their relationship uncertain when she left for Duke and he enrolled at the University of Tennessee. He had told his parents that he was going to date other girls, so she supposed she should be shopping around as well. But she couldn't see herself doing what the older girls at the orientation were telling her most girls did. On the other hand, what kind of social life would she have if she didn't? What kind of support would she find at a school that had replaced home? Those questions would dog her all year.

Some young women embrace, without much forethought, the freedom that is college life on most campuses today and end up being emotionally pummeled pretty badly. Victoria, willful by disposition and buoyed by her family and her family's religious faith, chose to sit out what passed as fun for many of her classmates.

I met her and Jocelyn immediately after the orientation. They had bonded the first week of school and would remain best friends all year, much like Nicole and Patty. Unlike Nicole and Patty, however, they were horrified by the hookup scene. With fewer than three weeks of school behind them, they already had tales to tell that first night over veggie pizza in a campus café.

Victoria began.

"Jocelyn and I were dancing together at a club. A guy came out on the floor with four girls and a few minutes later asked me for my phone number. So I gave it to him. Do you know he called me at one a.m. to ask if I wanted to hang out?"

Did she join him? I asked.

"Of course not!" she huffed, then continued, "A couple of nights later, another guy called me at three a.m. The next day a guy approached me and said I was the prettiest girl he had ever seen. 'The prettiest?' I replied. 'Do you ever watch TV?'"

Then it was Jocelyn's turn. A Washington, D.C.–area resident, she had had more experience with guys in high school than Victoria, but even she was shocked by the behavior of Duke students, male and female. "We know this girl who got drunk and showed up at a fraternity house at three a.m. asking for the baseball players," she began. "An upperclassman at the door told her they were asleep and ordered her to go back to her dorm. That girl, now, she roller skates with no brakes on."

"This morning, I saw a guy in my dorm leaving a girl's room wearing the same clothes and shoes that he had on the night before. Half of the guys here are predators. There's a black fraternity here and you know what we call it? NUPEs. That stands for 'Notorious Underground Pussy Eaters.'"

Like Victoria, Jocelyn was practicing the art of the quick retort. "A basketball player told me he could give me a sweet massage. I told him, 'And I can walk on your back.'"

These absolutely beautiful girls, both of them serious about organic chemistry and calculus, had decided that hooking up wasn't for them. I wondered to myself that September, with pheromones swirling like leaves on a brisk autumn morning, how long they could hold out. I called them separately a month later.

Jocelyn couldn't stop talking about a campus fashion show sponsored the previous night by the Black Student Alliance. It sounded a lot like the date auction Nicole and Patty had taken me to at GW, without the bidding.

"Me and Victoria walked in and saw this guy onstage and said, 'Oh my God, he's getting naked.' The guys were stripping down to their jock straps or G-strings. The girls were wearing camisoles and boy shorts. Everyone had their own little part, grinding onstage."

She said she didn't see any older adults there, although the lack of supervision didn't disturb her. "As long as no one broke anything, why should there be?" she asked.

In four weeks, she hadn't met anyone who appealed to her. "I see the guys here," she said, "and whatever they say to me, they're saying to other girls. I'm one of many, okay?" Clearly, being one of many wasn't going to be okay with her.

When I reached Victoria on the phone, I didn't hear the confident, somewhat bemused voice I had heard before. A call from Nicholas two weeks earlier had changed everything.

"Hi, Pook," he had said, and her heart skipped a beat as it always did when he used her pet name. They chatted about the upcoming parents' weekend, when he was supposed to visit, and she picked up some slight hesitation in his voice. Finally she asked him outright, "You *are* coming, right?"

"Well, no, I'm not," he said in his slow Tennessee drawl.

After several moments of silence, she couldn't hold back. "Why?"

" 'Cause we're not going to get back together."

Silence again. Then, from him, "I feel bad."

"Well, you should," she snapped and hung up.

She knew Nicholas's parents didn't like him dating a person of color. She also knew that long-distance relationships in college almost never last. When she thought about the call later, she realized that she had seen the split coming before she ever got to school. What she hadn't foreseen was how bleak her romantic options would be afterward.

"It feels hopeless when I think about the culture here," she said that day, sounding exactly the way Jamie would a few months later after she and Austin broke up. "Who am I going to find who really likes every aspect of me, who knows that I get my mustache waxed and that I have gross feet? Someone I can take a nap with and drool on his chest? The physical aspect of my relationship with Nicholas was a plus but by no means defined us."

It had taken Nicholas two months just to "pop kiss" her on the cheek, she said, and six more months passed before they decided to have intercourse. Now she was on a campus where "you go out expecting that [intercourse] is what you're going to do." She sighed. "If I start 'talking to' someone, he's not going to wait two months to make out. It's really hard to find someone to be patient and who respects you that much. In high school it was hard, but it's two or three times harder in college."

When she thought about Nicholas hooking up with someone at Tennessee, she felt sick. She was having trouble eating and sleeping, she said, and was pulling all-nighters because she couldn't concentrate and finish her homework at a reasonable hour. She was calling her mother two and three times a day.

Until this point, Victoria's life, like Jamie's, Nicole's and Cleo's, had been lovingly assembled by well-to-do parents with big dreams for their daughters and the means to help make those dreams come true. Nicholas's phone call had pulled the bottom out of their gilded cage, and Victoria was, for the moment, in free fall.

FROM *IN LOCO PARENTIS* TO ABSENTEE LANDLORD

College freshmen from privileged families go from prescribed course schedules and sports calendars to no schedules, from being restricted by V-chips and limited driving hours to no restrictions, from negotiating curfews with parents to setting their own hours. What to eat, what to study and whose bed to sleep in are only a few of the calls they make every day once they're on campus. For those who don't finish college, this free period before full-time employment may last only two or three years. But for those intent on at least a bachelor's degree, it lasts four to six years.

The feminist-inspired message of "You go, girl," embraced by devoted parents, follows them onto campus. They know they're supposed to do well in coursework but at first are confounded by the lack of rules telling them how to structure their academic life. Most of them quickly recover from this, however. They've had practice in high school taking tests and writing papers, and if they flounder, professors and advisers jump in to make sure they succeed, if for no other reason than to keep demanding parents away from the college gate.

Learning to navigate their personal freedom is a much lonelier undertaking. One of the most striking things about these years is the isolation in which students make decisions about their private lives. In high school, they're surrounded by parents and parents' friends, teachers and coaches, sometimes clergy and church youth leaders. They may not always seek out these adults to discuss the increasingly complicated choices they are making, but they know the grown-ups are there, and the grown-ups seek them out, at least occasionally.

Once new students arrive on a campus like Duke, the only older adults many see after orientation are their professors, and then only in class or for the occasional consultation about a paper or a grade. Over the last thirty years, as universities have demanded that professors spend more time doing research and getting published, faculty members have gradually removed themselves from the social life of the college and from their students.

At the same time, regulations governing dorm visits, behavior at campus functions and alcohol consumption either don't exist or go largely unenforced. Within the last couple of years, some universities, including Duke, have attempted to reinstate certain rules, particularly those governing underage drinking. But many students spend months, if not years, at college feeling both exhilarated and bewildered by the fact that, as columnist Katie Roiphe once put it, no one cares what they do anymore.

It was not always so. When this country was founded, new institutions like Harvard College were viewed as places where young men were prepared for leadership roles in the church, civil society and their families. Colleges were about moral as well as intellectual formation, and young charges labored under what one historian called "a virtual straitjacket of petty rules."

"Every possible aspect of student life was regulated," historian Frederick Rudolph writes, "promptness, attendance at classes and prayers, dressing, idling, fishing, gunning, dancing, drinking, fighting, gaming, swearing, and so on ad infinitum." And who enforced these rules? Faculty, he says, who were required to be "detectives, sheriffs, and prosecuting attorneys."

Colleges and universities continued to monitor student behavior, though with an increasingly lighter hand, up to the mid-twentieth century. Time and again, courts upheld a 1913 ruling that college authorities stood *in loco parentis,* or in place of the parents, when it came to the physical and moral welfare, as well as the mental training, of their students.

Then came the civil rights, women's and sexual liberation movements of the 1960s, as well as the Vietnam War and the protests it spawned. Students insisted that if eighteen-year-olds were old enough to do battle, they were old enough to enjoy the other privileges of adulthood. Whatever rights young men enjoyed, young women should enjoy as well. Society rather quickly accepted this logic, lowering to eighteen the age at which young people could vote, marry, make contracts and even purchase alcohol (in 1984, the legal drinking age was again set at twenty-one). And courts began to reject the idea that colleges had any obligation to protect students from harm or from harming each other. As Wendy White, senior vice-president at the University of Pennsylvania, explained, the courts held that "college is an educational, not a custodial, institution, and that it is both unrealistic and inconsistent with the objectives of higher education to hold institutions liable for injuries resulting from irresponsible student conduct."

Victoria's mother and father, who lived in their native Haiti during the 1960s and 1970s, were not a part of the rebellion that demolished *in loco parentis*. But the parents of many of today's students—and many college administrators themselves—took part in the demolition and continue to champion many of the freedoms it spawned. College students, they say, should be allowed to sample not only academic courses but dress and hair styles, drinking and dance routines, ways of flirting, sleep times, sleep places and sleep partners. The list is a long one, the theory being that if students are free to make their own choices, they ultimately will learn to make the right ones. This presumes that in their earlier years, parents gave them enough latitude to make mistakes, as well as an emotional and moral foundation sufficient to help them recover and learn from their failure.

The results of this freedom, on all but the most religious campuses, can boggle the minds of older adults who grew up in more regimented times. Core course requirements are looser, and students are given more ways in which to meet them. Students may design their own majors and take many courses pass/fail. In their time outside class, they can choose to invite anyone to their rooms at any hour, perform shows on campus that involve stripping down to almost nothing and slip considerable amounts of alcohol into parties unremarked.

The pendulum may be beginning to swing back, particularly when it comes to underage drinking. A recent Harvard study reported that one out of three colleges now bans alcohol on campus for any student, including those twenty-one and older. Fraternities have been eliminated on some small campuses such as Colby and Middlebury Colleges. Duke officials announced in 2006 that beginning in fall 2007, they would take the unprecedented step of limiting the amount of alcohol allowed at student tailgate parties preceding and following sports events—one element of a new Campus Culture Initiative spearheaded by Duke president Richard Brodhead.

Brodhead's action followed a well-publicized incident in March 2006, in which a young single mother hired to strip for an off-campus party was allegedly accosted and insulted by several drunk lacrosse players, three of whom were charged with rape. The alleged victim was black, the lacrosse players white, and the case immediately attracted national and international attention. The lacrosse players, or "laxers" as they were known on campus, mounted a vigorous defense. Whatever the outcome of the case would be, some faculty and students said the drinking and sex-infused culture it revealed had come to characterize much of Duke's social life.

To be fair to colleges like Duke, restricting student behavior can be a no-win situation. The lacrosse players' party, for example, took place in a private home off campus—with no college authorities anywhere around. This may have contributed to the rowdy, out-of-control atmosphere that no one at the party denied. Had the party taken place a decade earlier, when more students, including athletes, lived on campus, the behavior might have been different. But students left campus housing over the last few years because Duke administrators gradually made it more difficult for students to drink there. The houses into which they moved gave them more freedom to do as they pleased.

DEALING DATING THE FINAL BLOW

It is safe to say that dating would not have vanished completely, nor hooking up become as common as a cold, were it not for coed dorms and unrestricted visiting hours. For adolescents thinking about having sex, opportunity matters—a lot.

In the late 1980s, several colleges and universities tried to enact new codes limiting visitors in campus housing to certain hours while keeping coed dorms. Boston University led the effort, reporting that shortly before the rules went into effect, in a random check of dormitories over one week, 4,500 overnight visitors had been counted. BU president John Silber argued that an anything-goes policy infringed on the rights of students who needed privacy and that curfews did a couple of things. A new policy would prevent a student from entertaining a visitor night after night in front of his or her roommate or banishing the roommate to another room. And, if applied equally to guys and girls (unlike the old restrictions), it would give all students an easy excuse to exit uncomfortable situations.

BU's policies, although met with widespread protests by faculty as well as students, encouraged a few other institutions to impose similar regulations. Most schools, however, rejected the reforms. Administrators and faculty argued that coeducational living facilitates friendship between the sexes, teaching young women and men to get to know each other as people first, potential mates second. Many still say that. Jill Ringold, a health educator at Washington University in St. Louis, where most dorms are coed on each floor, told me, "There will always be some dormcest [what students call sex between couples living in the same dorm], but eventually they stop seeing each other as potential hookup material. Coed living doesn't encourage more sex."

Not all educators agree. Vigen Guroian, a professor of theology at Loyola College in Baltimore, harshly and publicly criticized his college and most other schools for having, as he wrote in one magazine article, "forfeited the responsibilities of *in loco parentis* and gone into the pimping and brothel business." He cites some of his female students as saying they feel pressured to hook up. One student depicted college as "an amusement park" of sex; another said "the peer pressure and the way things are set up make promiscuity practically obligatory." And this at a school where dorms are single-sex by floor and visitation is restricted—a more regulated environment than at many other colleges and universities.

Students I talked to, while not wanting tough restrictions restored, admitted there are advantages to limitations on opportunity. Leah, at Brown University, was one. Writing about the new girlfriend she met overseas, in a dorm where sexual activity was expressly forbidden, she said, "If we had been in the States, we'd probably have had sex and never gotten to know each other. Here, instead of finding out how to make each other come, we found out what makes each other tick."

Teresa, a vivacious, dark-haired sophomore at GW who was born in Venezuela and spent her early adolescence there, made a similar comparison. In Caracas, she said, young people live with their parents until they marry or find a well-paying job. As a result, they go out on dates as a matter of course.

She was surprised when she got to GW how different things were in this country. She didn't date at all her freshman year. At the beginning of sophomore year, she went on a date with a classmate in her political science course and the two of them received so much grief from their friends that they never went out again. Shortly thereafter, she started hooking up with a guy who lived down the hall in her dorm. Following a couple of evenings together, he told her that hooking up was all he wanted. A relationship was out of the question. "Why wouldn't he want to be my friend?" she asked me plaintively.

At the time of this interview, she was still steaming from being briefly "sexiled." She had returned to her dorm room from a campus job on Friday night around eight, exhausted. She turned the door handle and realized the door was locked. She could hear the sounds of her roommate and her roommate's boyfriend getting it on inside.

She knocked. And knocked. And dialed her roommate's cell phone, listening to it ring. She needed to go to the bathroom. She wanted to go to bed. Her roommate knew she worked from four to eight. Couldn't she have found another time for sex? It was not as if this evening was her roomie's first opportunity. She had had this boyfriend for two years.

Teresa sat out in the hall for half an hour until her roommate opened the door, offering only, "I was indisposed."

Recalling these and other stories, Teresa summarized her feelings: "You wake up one day and say, 'I'm sick of this. I'm hooked-up out.' "

In students' minds, dating is unnecessary if you're in each other's company all the time. As one of my GW students said, "We study together and live together, so we feel we don't need to date to get to know each other. And the beds are just a short walk away from the party."

And what pads they have in which to party. Hoping to woo to their campuses the brightest of the coddled generation, universities have begun to offer their own version of the comforts of home: two-, three- and four-bedroom apartments with private baths, kitchens, living rooms, swimming pools, hot tubs, high-speed Internet access, flat-screen TVs and cable, including HBO. These campus living quarters, paid for by Mom and Dad, are becoming so desirable that some juniors and seniors are asking to stay on campus rather than move off, a trend that would have been unheard of as recently as ten years ago.

Dates used to be a welcome escape from the eight-by-ten-foot cell you shared with another person of the same sex with whom you might or might not have anything in common. Today's students need no such alternative; they live with friends they've chosen in dorms that are splendid places to relax and have sex.

Emily, an easygoing, red-headed junior I taught at GW, recalled for us one evening what it was like to date in Dublin. As in Washington, bars are where young adults in Dublin hang out, and she made friends with several guys over pints of Guinness. Here's what was different: Irish universities do not provide housing, and students usually cannot afford to rent apartments. "So all the twentysomething guys I met lived at home and didn't have easy access to places for sex. I kind of liked that because I could let a guy hit on me without worrying about what would happen later."

FREEDOM OR PRESSURE?

Few reasonable people would argue that college students shouldn't be extended certain freedoms to find out what turns them on physically as well as intellectually. But certain questions follow: When does the freedom to have sex, for those who want it, turn into social pressure to have sex for those who don't? When does the freedom to strip onstage and dance provocatively in front of peers become exploitation of gender stereotypes? Is this the kind of liberal education that parents should be paying $45,000 a year for and, more important, the kind that campus authorities should be promoting?

I discussed these questions with GW's assistant athletic director shortly after the date auction. Mary Jo Warner was the university's representative the night that Morgan and other barely clad freshman athletes shimmied drunk on the catwalk in front of an audience of horny upperclassmen. Warner admitted that the event made her uncomfortable. "If I had a daughter, I wouldn't want her out there," she said. "It's on the edge."

Almost as an afterthought, she added, "The coaches stay way away from it."

She rationalized the university's support this way. The event raised about $1,000 for charity. (That was half of the proceeds; another $1,000 went to the sponsoring Student Athlete Advisory Council.) Second, the university assumes that student-run organizations should be given lee-way to decide what kind of activities they put on and how they will run those events.

"Some of the kids act as bouncers," she continued. "One year a guy got all greased up and opened up his pants. The bouncers peeled him off the stage. Occasionally, they'll glance over at me to see my reaction to something. I've told them if we get any complaints, they may have to stop it." So far, there had been none, according to Warner—which may mean only that few parents knew anything about it. None of the participants and young observers I talked to that night had ever mentioned the sub-ject of the auction to Mom or Dad.

While there is plenty of opportunity for sex in high school, too, even when adults are around and restrictions are in place, kids still have to re-turn home at some point on most days, and sometimes they get caught, forcing conversations with parents. The opportunities students have for sex at college, on the other hand, are unlimited, the opportunities to talk about their sexual experiences with older adults totally voluntary. By college, more of them are engaging in intercourse—nine out of ten by senior year compared with six of ten by senior year in high school. They are maturing intellectually to the point where they are beginning to re-alize that sex is not just the fun-and-games they once thought it was. Some want to talk, but they have no idea how to find someone to talk to.

Increasing opportunities for such discussion certainly couldn't hurt. Vu Le, a male columnist for the student newspaper at Washington Uni-versity in St. Louis, touched on this just after his girlfriend broke up with him:

"I am amazed that there is no academic course or guidance in that all-important area, the Romantic Relationship," he wrote in an issue of the university's *Student Life* newspaper, dubbed "Stud Life" by students. "College students are probably most concerned about two things: finding the right career and finding the right person. There are plenty of resources for the former. Unfortunately, for the latter, there is practically nothing."

Lest they be seen as moralistic preachers, college authorities have confined their oversight to physical—as opposed to physical and emotional—hazards. This is particularly true of sex. As Le pointed out, opportunities for instruction in the mechanics of sex are plentiful, but conversations about the context and aftermath of sexual relationships are not. This is in part because college authorities, like parents, are frequently uncomfortable talking about the negative, as well as positive, emotions of intimacy. So they put the entire responsibility on students to figure things out for themselves.

The health counseling service at Le's school is typical. The department runs an outstanding series of sessions each year about sex and maintains an easily accessible website with the latest information on contraception and communication. During one health service–sponsored Sex Week, the theme was "Raise the Bar . . . Communicate or Masturbate." The goal, according to the website, was to promote safer sex by encouraging students "to talk to partners about what they want from sexual activities." (Tellingly, the initiative was in response to students who said they needed information on sexual health more than they needed the then-current program on stress management.) The program carried the typical disclaimer that "many students choose not to be sexually active," but it was obviously aimed at those who do so choose. "Hooking up is part of the culture," health educator Jill Ringold told me. "My job is to find a way to make it healthier. That will also make it sexier."

Le referred to such courses in his column:

Sometimes we have visiting speakers, such as Dr. Ruth or the Dating Doctor. Sometimes there are forums on various topics concerning sex. The rest of the time we are forced to rely on our friends' bad experiences, our own bad experiences, or the pages of magazines like *Cosmopolitan* and, uh, *Maxim*.

None of these resources is scientific, and even if they were, a 90-minute forum or article on "how to achieve orgasm" cannot resolve all the complexities of relationships. What we need is at least a three-credit class on forming, sustaining, and terminating romantic relationships.

A few colleges and universities have started offering the kind of class Le was asking for: Ball State in Indiana, Pepperdine in California and Seattle Pacific in Washington, for example. But very few. As Marline Pearson, a college teacher in Madison, Wisconsin, who lobbies for such courses, notes, young women "have no 'North Star' for their intimate lives. By that, I mean no vision or expectation for good love, meaningful sex, commitment, marriage or father importance. They have received little guidance on how to build quality relationships, and even worse, they have no vision of quality relationships."

None of this means that colleges and universities stand idly by as their students drink themselves under the table and copulate like bunnies. Recent concerns across the country about campus safety, sexual assaults and lawsuits have, if nothing else, moved institutions to rethink their relationships with students when it comes to personal behavior. Somewhere between assuming the role of parent and assuming the role of bystander is the concept of providing "reasonable care." Administrators and faculty struggle with how they can demonstrate such care when they must both demand adherence to certain general standards of behavior and allow students to work out the details.

Physical safety is the first area they usually tackle; Duke's buses and

GW's vans, which provide round-the-clock transportation to and from dorms and other campus buildings, are examples of that. Many colleges and universities now also offer at least one substance-free dorm—where the use of illegal drugs, including alcohol, is grounds for removal. Overall alcohol consumption, which contributes heavily to the hookup scene, has proven far more difficult to monitor, and until very recently, college authorities did very little, calling their hands-off approach pragmatic. College students are going to drink, they reasoned, and it is safer for them to drink on campus than off. This was the argument Duke administrators used until recent years to allow kegs on campus.

And it was essentially the reason an administrator gave a parent for an annual event at Washington University in St. Louis called WILD. This acronym, the parent learned to his dismay, was short for "Walk In, Lie Down," a rock festival in the middle of campus that boasted free beer from hundreds of kegs. The beer maker, Anheuser-Busch, which is headquartered in St. Louis, would park delivery trucks of Budweiser just outside campus on this special Saturday night. After parents questioned this practice, the college administration banned kegs—but told students twenty-one and older they could each bring in a six-pack.

Generational experts Neil Howe and William Strauss say this generation is more willing than their parents were to accept such restrictions and, in fact, expect institutions to take care of them. When asked who's going to improve the schools, clean up the environment and cut the crime rate, for example, young people place more faith than older adults that it will be teachers, government and police. "They expect that people in those professions, hired by society to perform those critical social missions, should and will do their jobs," Howe and Strauss write, predicting that colleges may eventually reinstate more rules governing behavior, their decision driven partly by student expectations or, at the least, their acquiescence.

One of the few places on campus where young women can have the kind of conversations student columnist Le was talking about are women's centers such as the one at Duke. (Young men have no such places, although some centers, such as Duke's, invite men to join the women from time to time.)

The best of the centers attempt to be a sanctuary where young women of various beliefs and backgrounds can figure out what kind of relationships they want and how to achieve them. Such centers occasionally are run by women who make some of their more moderate feminist students—who may believe in abstinence, for example, or who may not be gay activists—uncomfortable. The staff who managed the Women's Center at Duke tried hard to make every woman comfortable, and during Victoria's freshman year helped sponsor two programs that strengthened Victoria's resolve to remain celibate as she recovered from her breakup with Nicholas.

Victoria's mother, Marie, says her second-oldest daughter always had a mind of her own. She has plenty of stories to prove it: Victoria at age two pouring a brand-new box of Cheerios all over the kitchen floor, immediately after her mother had told her not to; Victoria at three smearing petroleum jelly on her hair and her bedspread while Marie was bathing Victoria's sister; Victoria at five throwing Marie's keys in the garbage and not telling anyone, even after Marie searched all over the house.

"At one point I told my husband, 'I hate this child,' " Marie admits with a laugh, sounding exactly like Nicole's mom.

Marie and her husband, Albert, had created a remarkable life for their children under unusual circumstances. They had met at Cabrini Medical Center in New York City when Marie, then nineteen, was hospitalized after a car accident and Albert, twenty-seven, was a physician-in-training. They had dated for only six months when Albert, preparing to move to

Johnson City to start an internal medicine residency, asked Marie to marry and accompany him. He promised he would make enough money to give her a comfortable life and enable her to stay home and raise their children. Marie, the daughter of a wealthy coffee planter who had lost everything when the family moved to the United States, said yes, and they eloped.

Albert made good on his promise. When Victoria was three and her sister Andrea seven, he moved the family into a 1920s, antebellum-style mansion on four acres of rolling hills just inside the city limits. He and Marie had two more kids, and Marie, a spirited woman with a penchant for bright clothes and dangling earrings, became a homemaker and care-taker extraordinaire.

She restored and furnished the mansion to its original splendor. She dressed little Victoria in expensive smocked dresses and Italian leather shoes. She put all four children in private schools and brought them lunches of boiled shrimp, fruit and sandwiches she made on French bread. She served dinner every night at a twelve-seat Honduran ma-hogany table dressed with linen place mats and Limoges china, and threw parties for her children's friends around the large outdoor pool behind the house, serving the Haitian cuisine she quickly became famous for.

She steered her children away from African-American children, con-sidering the local families low-class and lacking ambition. Victoria adopted this attitude and did not have a single black friend in high school. It was only after she arrived at Duke that she met dark-skinned girls like herself from upper-income families and began to think of herself as black as well as Haitian.

She already thought of herself as a physician. From the time she could remember, she had followed her dad around, fascinated by what he did for a living. He, enchanted by her curiosity, took her with him to medical meetings and, as she got older, arranged work for her at the local hospital. Of all the girls I observed, her relationship to her father was the strongest by far, and suggested to me, as I reflected back on our year together, one reason why Duke's unhooked culture didn't unhook her.

Another key reason was the relationship she observed between her parents. Like many young women I had interviewed, she dreamed of being it all: a physician, a mother and a wife. But unlike the other women, she wanted a marriage that looked exactly like her parents'. She had watched them closely, if surreptitiously, over the years, and envied the little things they seemed to enjoy doing together. Late at night in bed, they talked, cuddled and watched TV. Marie rose at five a.m. every day just to prepare coffee for Albert before he went to work. Albert would do anything Marie asked of him, though he'd sometimes grumble.

She realized that should she become a doctor, she wouldn't have the time to devote to a husband that her mother did. But she was sure she could build a similar union using different materials, provided she could feel, and find, the same devotion.

"Of course my parents argue sometimes, that's normal," she said. "But he's the only one for my mom, and she's the only one for him." Here it was again, a reminder that girls, like guys, learn how to love, care for and be sexual with a partner first by what they see at home. I heard this from each girl in this book, dropped casually in conversations, little details about how their parents did or did not make time for each other, did or did not play with each other, did or did not express affection for each other, did or did not negotiate differences well.

Only one cloud hung stubbornly over Victoria's teenaged years: her body. It was of almost classic, hourglass proportions, maintained by a vigorous running schedule. But Victoria thought her legs and behind, in particular, were too big, and a boyfriend in ninth grade didn't help matters. He called her "jiggly butt" and once said to her, "Just think what you'd look like if you stopped running." She knows now that she should have dropped him immediately, but she dated him from March of ninth grade until he broke up with her in July. Even after that, his words stuck with her and she dieted all through high school, confining lunch during her senior year to a can of Slim-Fast. To this day, every time she eats a brownie she pictures it settling immediately in her thighs.

Nicholas, however, thought she was beautiful. His father worked for a packaging company; his mother was a homemaker. Though he wasn't a country boy, he had the unruly shock of brown hair, tall frame and natural good looks of a country-western star. He played baseball at the high school that Victoria had transferred to in ninth grade. She first approached him in their junior year, asking him to a formal dance. He accepted and they went to the dance together, but he did not immediately pursue her, so she pursued him. They started dating seriously after Valentine's Day that year and didn't stop until they went off to separate colleges. Eight months into their relationship they had sex, even though she had told herself she would wait until marriage. Part of the reason she changed her mind, she suspects now, is that nearly all her friends had already had sex in ninth or tenth grade. She also thought it was just possible that she might marry him and went around the house humming one of their favorite songs, Shania Twain's "Forever and for Always."

Nicholas was a frequent visitor in Marie's kitchen, always happy to find a piece of cherry or blueberry "pah," as he called it. Marie welcomed him but didn't think he was husband material for her daughter. He displayed little ambition and said he'd be content to come back to Johnson City after college. "Victoria has bigger fish to fry," Marie told me. She told Victoria the same thing, but Victoria, ever the hardhead, refused to listen.

Marie said she knew that Victoria and Nicholas had slept together, even in her house. "It's not what I would have wanted for her," she said. "But at least it was within a relationship. I've always told my girls I don't want them to be sluts. If they're going to sleep with a man, it should be in a relationship." She saw a resemblance between Victoria's first love and her own, she told me one afternoon as we were sitting in her large, comfortable kitchen overlooking the backyard patio, swimming pool and mountains. In her late teens in New York City, she had been in love with, and lost her virginity to, a gorgeous boy. She dated him for three years, even as, later on, he cheated on her. She had told Victoria this story and warned her that she might have fallen in love with the act of sex with Nicholas rather than with Nicholas himself. Victoria listened but insisted that it was not her story.

Victoria arrived at Duke on her first day in a big black Navigator that her dad had given her. The SUV virtually swallowed her up, and a campus of 5,000-plus undergraduates threatened to do the same. But she was determined not to let that happen and sought out the help Duke offered.

She moved onto the freshman-only East Campus, a collection of colonial-style brick buildings on either side of two huge grass circles known as The Yard. In 1995, Duke administrators had decided to sequester freshmen from worldlier upperclass students, a decision that is still debated. Victoria signed up to live in the substance-free dorm. "The people there were no fun," she recalled. "They never went out or said 'Hi' to me in The Yard unless I said 'Hi' first." One week after moving in, she asked to transfer to a regular dorm.

She declared a pre-med major and enrolled in intense subjects like chemistry that required three hours of classroom time every week plus four hours in the lab. She landed a role in *The Vagina Monologues*, knowing that rehearsals would consume what little free time she had.

"I don't have time for boys," she told me in January with a certain degree of satisfaction. The closest she came to socializing with guys was going to clubs and campus parties on weekends with Jocelyn and other girlfriends. Most of the time, she danced with the girls but on occasion she would agree to accompany a guy to the dance floor, insisting that they dance in the old-fashioned way facing each other, several inches apart.

Her dislike for her body, as inexplicable as it might seem to outsiders,

continued to be a problem. Early rehearsals for the *Monologues* reminded
her of this when the codirector asked each cast member to name three
things they liked about their bodies. "He insisted I try, but I couldn't think
of three," she said. Given this insecurity, Nicholas's departure made her
vulnerable to any halfway decent–looking guy who made a pass at her.
She knew this, and embraced her role in the *Monologues* as not only a time
filler but a reminder that her body was something special, not something
to give away to just anyone.

On the night of the *Monologues*, she appeared onstage in a sleeveless,
silk pink-and-orange nightgown to deliver the soliloquy "Reclaiming
Cunt." She was playing a woman in Pittsburgh who had decided to claim
the c-word as her own, thereby ridding it of its pejorative connotation.

"I call it cunt," she said, a short, lone figure under a spotlight. With
each line, her normally soft voice grew louder. "I proclaim it—cunt! I
really like it. Listen to it. Cuh, ca, cover, cackle . . ." She pronounced each
letter individually, making new words, all the while sliding her hands seductively over her torso, waist, hips and thighs.

She got to the T. "Tendril, time, tell me . . . Tell me . . . cunt!"

The stage went dark and the audience, which included her sister Andrea, applauded loudly. Like other girls in the performance, she floated
on that roar of the crowd for days afterward.

Her biggest boost came from Duke's Baldwin Scholars program,
named for the first dean of what was known years earlier as the Women's
College. The scholars, eighteen freshman girls chosen from among
seventy-five applicants, were part of what Duke administrators called "an
alternative social environment." The scholars were guided by faculty
members to "develop their own identities, set their own standards and
learn leadership skills," in short, to enjoy some of the advantages of
single-sex education within a coeducational setting. The inaugural class
began in the second semester of Victoria's freshman year. Scholars attended a seminar twice a week, went on a mountain retreat and met var-

ious women executives on and off campus. (A year later, in 2005–2006, they began living together.)

The program, which grew out of Duke's Women's Initiative, had its critics. Some asked what it said about a college when the only way a considerable number of girls at that college could feel supported was to remove themselves from it. Some said that the money and energy going into the scholars' program would be better spent improving relationships between female and male students campuswide.

But it was a godsend for Victoria, as protected as she had been growing up. Among other things, it helped reinforce her decision not to date or hook up, for although some of the other scholars did both, they encouraged her not to until she was ready. Unlike Nicole's girlfriends, or Sienna's, these girls were already sure enough of themselves to know that not everyone had to act the way they did. "When you're in a serious relationship, you are tempted to define yourself by that other person," one girl told Victoria during the second semester. "You need to spend time with yourself, figure out what your strengths are."

That was good for her to hear because over winter break in Johnson City, she felt she had slid backward where Nicholas was concerned. She had run into him at a party, accompanied him to his older brother's apartment and, as she put it, "messed around." The next day, she was disappointed in herself. They had told each other that night that they didn't want to be in a relationship. So what *were* they? He asked her over to the apartment several more times during the almost monthlong vacation, and although she went, she didn't sleep with him. When she was tempted to do more than kiss, she remembered how much pain she had suffered her first semester when she had lost him as a steady boyfriend.

On several evenings, they watched *The Best of Will Ferrell* and other DVDs and played Nintendo sitting on opposite ends of the couch. One night she asked him if he had hooked up with any girls at UT.

"What do you mean 'hook up'?" he replied.

"Have sex," she said.

He admitted he had kissed a girl, "but that was all."

He then asked her the same question.

She hesitated so she could see him squirm, then told him no.

In March, on her nineteenth birthday, she spent most of the day cry-ing because, as she told me, "I'm now thinking it's not plausible for us to be together, but I'm still not over him." She refused to give in to drink-ing during times like these and used Jocelyn's ear as a support instead. She also turned to her Bible.

Very late in our year together, she revealed that she and her family were Jehovah's Witnesses, a Christian organization founded in the nine-teenth century that stresses Bible study and strict adherence to biblical rules. When she was home, she attended Sunday-morning services. At Duke, she kept a Bible by her bed and every night followed a routine that reduced her anxieties:

"I wash my face, brush my teeth, read the daily Scripture message and then a little on my own from the Bible.

"My faith doesn't keep me from hooking up," she said in response to a question, "but it reinforces my decisions not to."

Well over half of college students, when surveyed, say that religion is important to them. One-third see their university as a possible place for exploring their spiritual side. These proportions are up from a decade ago. A similarly significant jump has been noted among high school kids, with the biggest rise occurring not among those with little money and ambition—the stereotyped believers—but among young achievers who anticipate finishing four years of college. While there are assuredly many reasons for this interest, the number one reason that young faith-ful give is their "direct personal relationship with the Divine," says Brad Wilcox, a University of Virginia sociologist who has spent years re-searching the subject. "Their brains are changing, their relations with family, friends and the opposite sex are changing, [and] we know that people often turn to God in the midst of momentous changes. Adolescents are no different."

A national study of young people, religious and secular, in which Wilcox was involved, concluded what Victoria could have told the researchers: that students of faith are less likely to be depressed, less likely to smoke, drink and have sex, and more satisfied with their families and school. This leaves one wondering whether after all the ambitious child-rearing that parents of this generation of students have done—all the Discovery toys, Suzuki piano lessons, four a.m. swim practices, SAT practice classes and summer camps in faraway places—they might have done as well or better and saved a lot of money by just taking their kids to church, temple or mosque.

Once they get to campus, students like Victoria must apply their faith to their sexual lives largely on their own because in the area of religion and sexuality, as in other areas of their personal lives, older adults on campus either take extreme positions or refrain from starting such conversations. Donna Freitas, a religious studies teacher at St. Michael's College in Colchester, Vermont, spoke to this point in a column for *The Wall Street Journal*.

Religious conservatives on campus preach abstinence and advocate virginity pledges whose overall impact is negligible, she wrote, and liberals talk only about sex and not religion.

So [students] wander, unmoored and often unhappy, through all the pleasure-possibilities that unsupervised campus life can offer them. Yet they never feel quite free of the ethical grounding—often religious in character and instruction—of their upbringing. . . . My students are crying out for spiritual conversation. In the safety of like-minded company, they also admit to wanting more from their relationships than just sex. Yet the gap between these cravings and sexual extravagance is wide.

The number one reason young people get in the habit of going to church is because their parents take them. Victoria's mom, Marie, had done that. And Victoria, with help from her mother, had negotiated a spiritual compromise with her sexuality that at the moment seemed to be working. Her religion prohibited sex before marriage. She had ignored that prohibition but only with someone she deeply loved. More important to her was her religion's view that marriage was a one-time-only arrangement sanctioned by God. This gave her pause. Would she ever find a worthy person? The choices she had encountered at Duke didn't look promising.

We talked about this on her next-to-last day of school over lattes in a campus coffee shop. We had run into a male friend of hers, and after he left, she told me that this friend had a fraternity brother "who will not leave me alone. It's just because he wants to get in my pants. Guys here expect you'll do whatever, and that's not the kind of girl I am. If they think I'm a prude, then they're clearly not worth my time."

She was proud of not having hooked up once all year. Nor had she dated, for fear her date would want to hook up. The problem, of course, was that she therefore had no one to compare Nicholas to, no one against whom she could test her experiences with, and feelings for, Nicholas. She had not given up hope of finding that person, however.

"Sometimes," she said, "I think to myself, If sex was that good with Nicholas, imagine what it will be like with my husband after fifteen years."

But how would she find that husband? I asked myself. As strong-willed as she was in some areas of her life, she didn't yet feel certain enough of herself to seek out a new relationship that could be on her terms. In fact, she didn't, at least in our year together, even see the possibility of such a relationship.

I gave her credit for realizing she wasn't ready. This is an important legacy that feminism has left with this generation. The wisest feminists say to young women: Listen to yourselves. There is no lasting satisfaction in taking a man to bed and leaving him at will, just because you can or because your friends tell you to. Very little good comes of sleeping with a guy, or even making out with a guy, you barely know. If you're interested in a guy, study him as you would for an exam. Spend time with him. Allow him to get to know you.

Shaida learned these lessons the hard way, on her own. Many girls do. Like Cleo, they grow up in families that appear to show more interest in their school lives than in their personal lives. They pick up early on parental expectations that they should give 110 percent to everything they do. They do a lot, and their parents make sure that they have everything they need in the way of material goods, expert assistance and a safe environment in order to perform up to their potential. They come to expect perfection, or as near to perfection as they can achieve, in everything they do.

The problem is, relationships are never perfect. Additionally, relationships take time and effort, and girls have little of either. So rather than settle for a relationship that is maybe sixty percent terrific, girls hook up beginning in high school because it's the only activity they can possibly manage and comes with no great expectations. By the time they get to college, hooking up may have become their definition of a relationship, and much of the college environment supports it. Some, like Cleo, discover longer-lasting attachments but even then find themselves hooking up on the side. We are only beginning to see the possible implications.

Hooking Up: Why It Matters

ALICIA'S STORY

"Will we be able to find someone we trust for a lifetime?
Will we be likely to stick around and work out problems?"
—ALICIA, TWENTY

licia arrived at Duke in the fall of 2002, tall and slender with straight, shoulder-length black hair and the graceful movements of a gazelle. She had made a name for herself at her public high school as a covaledictorian, award-winning gymnast, church youth group leader and Sunday school teacher. With all her accomplishments, she was very much like the other young women there.

But she was also very different. She had been born in Korea to Korean parents and adopted as an infant by an American couple who brought her back to the Washington, D.C., suburb where she grew up. Her father and mother were a loving, strict, conservative Christian couple who seemed never to know quite what to do with a daughter who could be alternately meek and headstrong, solicitous and morose. She did not get along with them particularly well—or with the brother and sister who came along after her—during much of her adolescence. She spent much of her time in high school in the company of a couple of friends.

Her family lived on the modest income of her father, so she went to Duke on a partial scholarship and took a job on the salad line of the cafeteria to help pay for books and supplies. On a campus where many girls came from wealthier families, her feeling of being unlike those she knew increased.

She was a junior at Duke when I observed her, and majoring in civil engineering. It was her "apartness" that helped convince me I should make her the subject of the book's final section. That, and her ability, extraordinary at her age, to make observations about her classmates and culture that were precisely on point. Watching and listening to her, I was reminded of the technique Woody Allen used as Alvy Singer in the movie *Annie Hall,* turning to viewers and explaining the truth of what was taking place around him.

Hooking up offers girls the opportunity to exert their independence, explore their sexual desires and capabilities and try to keep their emotional lives under control. But some experts in the field of adolescence, even as they acknowledge the upsides, say hooking up can also act as an obstacle to real intimacy, which they call the hallmark of a satisfying adult life. They see potential for long-term dangers to young women and young men—physical, emotional and practical—if hooking up comes to define a way of being.

Near the end of my research I was posing tough questions to these experts as well as to young women, and watching Alicia live out much of what I was hearing about. This section reflects the thinking of those specialists, with Alicia as both subject and key witness to their concerns.

From the time she was in high school, Alicia never spent more than two weeks without a guy. But that's not to say she was promiscuous. Holding hands was as far as she went with anyone until her first kiss at seventeen, and she departed for college a virgin.

As a freshman at Duke, she fell in love with a student at the University of Virginia whom she had met at home during the summer that had just ended. She had sex with him and continued to see him until the following April, when they broke up. Then she embarked on a series of sexual and romantic encounters that lasted two years, until midfall of the year I was with her. Two of those attachments lasted several months each, but most were much shorter, including one with a well-known actor that lasted all of one night.

He was a lecturer in his thirties, and her friends dared her to hook up with him. At a party that followed his evening talk, she struck up a conversation, and eventually the two of them found a private room at the restaurant, where they made out heavily. He asked her to accompany him to his hotel room but she declined, telling me later that that was "way too sketchy. I got what I came for, including a good story to tell."

"It was the most exhilarating hookup I'd ever had," she added.

One advantage a young woman enjoys today, which past generations of women did not, is that when someone catches her interest, she can do more than bat her eyelashes, tip her cigarette for a light or wait for days while he works up his nerve to ask her out. Girls like Cleo, Nicole and Alicia thought nothing of approaching a guy directly, and that could feel really good. In a survey of 1,000 college women across the country, a sociologist at the University of Texas found that those who had hooked up reported a variety of emotions, including feeling "strong, desirable and sexy" as well as "awkward" and "hurt."

"It is fun sometimes to know that you can seduce someone," Alicia wrote to me in the beginning of our year together. "Who hasn't had a random fling or one of those hyperactive nights where you go out with your girls and have a good time attracting the attention of some random charming guy?"

Laurence Steinberg, a psychology professor at Temple University who specializes in adolescence, also sees some merit in the fact that because sex is not a big deal to many of these girls, they feel less obligated to a man simply because they've slept with him. Women who came of age in the 1950s and 1960s can certainly remember the expectation of obligation, imposed by parents and the culture at large, and how wrongheaded it felt. Steinberg suggests that today's young women, absent that burden, may be more confident than their mothers were in abandoning bad relationships and pursuing good ones. This may make them less likely to jump into marriages that don't make sense logistically or financially. Ashley Wilson, a senior at the College of William & Mary, in Virginia, and not a fan of hooking up, concedes this may be true: "Perhaps the gravity of 'commitment' hits home with girls of this generation better than it did in previous generations where women ended up in unhappy or unfaithful marriages."

THE DOWNSIDES, STARTING WITH DISEASE

Now let's consider the medical math. The more sexual encounters a girl has, the more chances she has to be infected with a sexually transmitted disease or get pregnant. Girls and young women know they can dodge the pregnancy bullet by sticking to blow jobs, but an alarming number of them, especially high school girls, think that will protect them from infection as well.

The pregnancy rate among girls aged fifteen to nineteen has decreased by about one-third since 1990, a large proportion of that decrease among black girls. The abortion rate has dropped as well. But the incidence of sexually transmitted disease (STD) remains stubbornly high—higher, in fact, in the United States than in any other developed country.

Although only slightly more than one in ten women report having an STD, almost nineteen million new cases, including HIV cases, are reported each year. And although fifteen- to twenty-four-year-olds represent only one-quarter of sexually active Americans, they make up nearly half of these new cases. More young women than young men now contract STDs, and the medical community's concerns have shifted from men in their late twenties to teenaged girls.

Physicians are particularly concerned about chlamydia, the most frequently reported sexually transmitted disease in the country, according to the Centers for Disease Control and Prevention. Three out of four cases of chlamydia occur in young people under age twenty-five. Some scientists estimate that by age thirty, one out of two sexually active women will show evidence of having had chlamydia—a particular worry because the disease, if untreated, can lead to infertility. Infertility rates are rising in this country, and several leading fertility experts project that the number of women trying unsuccessfully to conceive will double in the next decade, to about one in three.

So, in addition to worrying about whether her new partner will call the day after a tumble in the sack, or whether she is pregnant, a girl has to worry about how many other people he has slept with and whether he has given her a disease with lifelong implications that nothing, other than not having sex, could have absolutely prevented. She may also worry about how many people she sleeps with and whether she may be passing on a disease she doesn't yet know she has.

Several girls interviewed in this book were being treated for some kind of sexually related infection (and asked for confidentiality), and most of them knew at least one infected girl. Chlamydia, the human papillomavirus (HPV) and genital herpes, which can be transmitted by oral sex, anal sex or vaginal sex, were the infections they talked about most often. One young woman, late in our year together, told me she had been diagnosed with a dangerous strain of HPV, which makes her vulnerable to cervical cancer. "The scary thing is that the form of HPV I have is often undetectable in guys," she told me. "It's not just that they don't see symptoms but that tests can't find it. So even a past partner who tested clean could have given it to me."

Did she always insist on her partner using a condom in the past? I asked. Girls aged fifteen to nineteen report condom use more than any other age group, but even then, the proportion is only two out of five and declines in college. The young woman admitted that on a couple of occasions, she had not.

A girl can tuck a Trojan into her purse on a Saturday night, but there is no such device to protect her heart. William Beardslee, a psychiatry professor at Harvard University, says girls who hook up are too quick to believe they can simply decide not to get hurt. "The big issue for me is it's hard to believe true sexual intimacy is unconnected from personal intimacy," he said. "These young women need to be careful not to fool themselves."

Alicia agreed. "Your mind and heart don't split down the middle because your physiology connects the two," she wrote. "Think about it. When you are emotionally close to someone, you appreciate physical interactions with them. You hug your friends, kiss people on the cheek, link arms when you walk and lay your head on the shoulders of a guy friend when you're watching a movie. And when you are physically close to someone, you seek out emotional closeness, as much as you might fight against it."

She knew whereof she spoke. Shortly after she broke up with her freshman-year boyfriend, she slept with a guy she had known since high school. "Though he made the effort to be sweet and call me to make sure I got home safe, I never felt like more than an object to him," she wrote. In the summer after her freshman year, she went out for drinks after work with another guy she met in Washington and then went back to his apartment, where they made out a lot until his roommates arrived home. She saw him at work several times after that night, but he didn't talk to her, which was upsetting, she said.

"At that point I hadn't really mastered the attachment-free hookup."

Girls, more than guys, report feelings of love early in a relationship, particularly after they've had sex, and will go to great lengths to keep a relationship going. After a breakup, they also are more likely to report intense feelings of sadness, followed by depression that can emerge as late as half a year or more after the relationship ended. Alcohol abuse, eating disorders, even suicide can result, particularly if a girl has a family history of depression or if her depression goes untreated.

Says Susan Nolen-Hoeksema, a University of Michigan psychologist who researches depression, "Something about dating behavior and dating relationships can be toxic to girls' health."

Significantly, the shorter the relationship, the more likely depression will show up. Most hookups are nothing if not brief. This means that girls who hook up serially have to work very hard—harder than they may know or admit—to squash or deny natural feelings of connection, making themselves even more vulnerable to depression.

Consider also that if a girl initiates a hookup or hookup relationship and it bombs, she can't hold the guy completely responsible and may receive little sympathy from anyone, including her girlfriends. If she turns around and hooks up again, she takes little time to analyze what happened in the previous encounter or to recover from a disappointment she doesn't want to acknowledge. Like the driver who has an accident during rush hour, she may not see a place to pull over. "It's not so much that hookups happen, it's that nothing else happens," Alicia said. "You don't see a way out."

So there the young woman is, avoiding real relationships because they consume time, energy and emotions, and discovering to her surprise that hookups take just as much. Doubt becomes her constant companion, forcing her to ruminate on what she should have done. The most diffi-

cult, dissonant moment may come when a girl understands that by trying to take control, she has simply done to herself what she meant to prevent boys from doing to her. Alicia wrote:

> Most girls eventually realize that getting a guy to sleep with you is
> just a fancy way of "letting" a guy sleep with you. Guys aren't too
> picky about who they sleep with. You begin to ask yourself, are you
> like currency? It can be very taxing.
>
> You try so hard to stay free and unattached and indifferent while
> you attach yourself all the while, and then suddenly it's over and the
> emotions of every time in that relationship when you should have
> stood up for yourself or denied him something, all surface.
>
> Every time you weren't indifferent just pisses you off, and instead
> of being sad that you are hurt by the loss of someone (which ar-
> guably acknowledges your capacity to connect with someone, a pos-
> itive thing), you are angry that you let that person hurt you. And
> friends are quick to help you curse that bastard, which is easier than
> trying to heal your soul. This does two things: One, it glosses over
> the deep hurt/emotional wounds; and two, you experience it both as
> a relationship and as a hurtful battle with your attachment needs.
> Since it ends badly, you end up hating both your needs *and* rela-
> tionships in general.

Young women may be at greatest risk of emotional distress not in
high school but during the college years because many of them are living away from their families for the first time. Psychiatrist Richard Kadison, chief of mental health services at Harvard University, makes this
argument in his book *College of the Overwhelmed*, in which he describes
what he calls "an epidemic of depression" on campus. Kadison and other
professionals paint a disturbing picture. For every five young people
who reach twenty-four, one will have been diagnosed with major de-

pression. The percentage of students seeing college counselors for depression has doubled since the late 1980s. In 2005, more than two out of three college-aged women, and more than one out of two college-aged men, said they felt hopeless at least once during the past school year. Only somewhat fewer said they had felt so depressed, at least once, that it was difficult to function.

Kadison acknowledges that the growing proportion of students seeking help may reflect in part a greater willingness to admit their depressed feelings. Also, more students are in college with the help of medication after being treated for depression so severe that, in the past, colleges would not have admitted them. Of course, events other than failed relationships can precipitate distress: grades and exams, family troubles, financial worries. But right up there, says Kadison, is social pressure, including the pressure to have an active romantic and/or sexual life.

Depressed people tend to fall into two categories: those who avoid relationships and those who, governed by a powerful need to be cared for, try to stay in relationships at all costs. Sienna, the high school "player," spoke about the latter when she said, "You're doing something you know is really wrong and are incapable of stopping it. This sometimes leads to feeling sad."

Sienna's feelings of sadness were brief, as many girls' are. Alicia's lasted longer. Looking back on her pattern of hooking up in college, she realized:

> I was not able to leave guys when I knew I should because I was not
> confident that I would be okay without them. I think a lot of this goes
> back to the whole adoption thing, and being generally terrified of
> being hurt by people who deem me "not good enough to
> keep around."

Doing these things more often doesn't mean they get understood or interpreted differently, which is a point that seems to get lost. To

some degree all of my sexual encounters in the first three years of
college messed with my emotions and my opinions of myself. I felt
generally great when I had a guy I was interested in, and more and
more ecstatic as things started to fall into place. Then things would
fall apart and everything would suck tremendously. I'd question if I
was a worthy person and if I deserved love.

Even with boyfriends, as opposed to hookup partners, she said, "I wasn't
getting what I needed and couldn't speak up for myself because I was
afraid of being rejected, even by someone whom I didn't even like or
someone who was hurting me."

Like many college-aged women, she struggled with these emotions
almost entirely alone. When she was home on break, she visited a ther-
apist she had seen occasionally in high school. But she didn't feel comfortable revealing her discomfort to her parents or any but one or two
friends. Essentially, she was her sole source of support, assisted by a
journal in which she wrote every day.

The first day I stepped onto the Duke campus, I ate lunch on an outdoor
patio near the student center. A dozen or so young women and men sat
scattered at other tables, including three thin girls who spent most of the
time chatting while nibbling at salads that appeared to be mostly leaf let-
tuce. It may be that the salad munchers simply wanted to stay skinny;
after all, from the time they start school, girls pick up the message that
thin is in. But it was also possible that some of them were suffering
from anorexia.

In the United States, anorexia, or self-imposed starvation to lose
weight, affects 7 million women (and 1 million men), almost half of
whom start starving themselves between ages sixteen and twenty. Researchers estimate it claims the lives of ten percent of sufferers.

Sometimes, says Harvard's Kadison, anorexia is genetic or biological. But in other girls, it is a way of ordering a world that is uncertain. In college, he writes, "there are many overwhelming decisions to be made about academic courses, relationships, sexuality, values, future careers, and on and on. An anorectic can avoid making these decisions by blocking out everything around her and focusing intently only on her body size and on what she will eat and not eat each day."

Alicia did this beginning late in high school and on and off in college. Here is how she described her ritual:

> In high school, I would break everything into pieces before eating piece by piece. I'd count each bite and chew each piece at least twenty-five times. I could not eat more than half of anything in front of me. I stopped drinking calories (like soda, juice and milk). I stopped using sauces or condiments. I used diet pills to keep up my energy.
>
> In college, I stopped eating meals. Even now if I order takeout, it will usually make at least four meals. I started using the gym and couldn't leave the machine until all the people who were there before me were gone, and on multiples of five seconds I had burned a multiple of ten calories. I still didn't drink calories (unless they were alcohol).

"Once you've trained your mind," she added, "your habits linger."

Alicia never considered her disorder serious. At her thinnest she weighed 110 pounds; more often she was in the low 120s—plenty, she thought, for her five-foot-seven-inch frame.

At Duke, she said, her anorexia was a reaction to classmates who seemed to have so much more of everything in their lives, especially expensive clothes and money from home to spend on whatever they chose. "I didn't have those things and felt very much on the outs," she recalled, "and so my disorder came back as a way to prove to myself that I was superhuman, that I didn't need all those things that everyone else needed."

Her anorexia, she came to believe, was really about shrinking her world "into a very small and narrow space. If I could control everything in the world of food, my life would seem in balance." Hooking up, she suggested, could play a similar role in girls' lives. Since forming serious relationships seems so overwhelming, girls seek out something more confined that they think they can manage, only to discover that hooking up leaves them feeling less in control than ever. Which, of course, could lead them to anorexia.

Two events in the second half of her sophomore year damaged Alicia's fragile sense of self-control. The first involved her sorority formal. She had needed a date, and three sorority sisters suggested Kevin, a junior in the same fraternity as their dates. Fresh from breaking off a short-term relationship, Alicia was not interested in hooking up and assumed that Kevin wouldn't be, either, because he had a girlfriend at another school. She asked him to be her "platonic date" and he agreed.

Early in the evening, Alicia arrived at a friend's dorm and changed into fancy clothes. She left her jeans and a T-shirt in Kevin's room, and she and Kevin joined the three other couples at an off-campus apartment for food and booze. They arrived at the dance a bit drunk, although not "sloppy wasted," as she put it. At the end of the dance, Kevin accompanied her back to his room so she could pick up her clothes. They started to make out and she warned him that she didn't want to have sex.

His reply, she recalled, was: "Then give me a hand job."

She did, but before she could finish, he pushed her down flat on the couch and positioned himself on top of her.

"No. Stop," she said softly, but he ignored her, clamping his hand over her mouth. As she tried to turn away, he forced himself inside her. He was not wearing a condom. She tensed up and then tried to go numb, to mentally escape. "I watched it happening from above," she said. "I just wanted to detach from my body." He fell asleep afterward, and she left for her dorm "having this dirty feeling of not knowing what to do or who to tell or whether it was really my fault."

What upset her almost as much as the assault was Kevin's reaction over the next few weeks when he saw her on campus. He would nod and try to start a conversation as if nothing had happened. "It hurts to know he doesn't think he did anything wrong," she said in an e-mail six months after the assault.

In that same missive, which was eerily similar to the e-mail from Shaida months after her incident with the lacrosse player, Alicia mentioned another attack that had taken place only a few months before Kevin's. Pat was someone she barely knew; she met him at a party in her dorm. They drank and then went to her room, where they started stripping and making out. He asked her if she wanted a massage, but before she could answer, he climbed on top of her. He mumbled about getting condoms and she told him not to worry, that they weren't going to have sex. He kept trying to get inside her and she panicked, asking herself, How do I get myself out of this? Eventually he managed to force his penis into her mouth and start thrusting. Summoning what strength she had, she pushed him off, kicked him out of her room and ran into the shower, crying.

She and I met for coffee a couple of weeks after I received her confessional e-mail. When I asked her for details of the two incidents, she shrugged her shoulders and didn't respond. Had she reported what happened to campus authorities? I asked. No, she said, she had not. Why not?

"There's not much to say," she finally said in a voice so low I had to lean over the table to hear. "It happens to everyone, I guess." Over the next few months I would learn that she blamed herself for not saying no enough times or with enough force. "It's hard for me to understand that they did something wrong," she told me. "I considered them assaults, but . . . they fell into the gray area."

Oh, the gray area—that insidious "if I hadn't gone to that party" place, that "if I had only stopped after one beer" place, that "if I hadn't worn such a revealing top and come on to that hot guy" place where young women go when someone they probably know lays siege to their most private parts and everyone assumes it was at least partly their fault. More than half the time, they're drunk and can't remember details, and most of the time they don't press charges. The incident with Kevin was clearly rape, but some defense lawyers and even some students have taken to calling such episodes "gray rape" out of a mistaken belief that when both partners have been drinking heavily, responsibility for what happened falls into a gray area.

This is one of the most egregious, and least-talked-about, implications of the hookup culture. In gray rape, the girl who may have come on like a hunter becomes the hunted. Whose fault is that? For older generations, it seems clear that it's the guy's if she resists in any way or is drunk. Girls like Alicia and Shaida aren't quick to say that, so reluctant are they to see themselves as powerless. Faculty sponsors of the Duke report on gender, which looked at issues of security on campus, were surprised by the number of female students who wanted better protection from stranger rape (increased patrols in parking lots, for example) but were ambivalent about needing protection from their own classmates. "Students expressed both support and blame for students victimized by acquaintance rape," the report said.

My students at GW, most of them female, engaged in a lively discussion around this question and were, in fact, the ones from whom I first heard the phrase "gray rape." A couple of students supported the current legal standard. Revealing clothes, stiletto heels, flirtation and making out are not an invitation to an open house, they said. Guys know when they're stepping over the line.

Most of the students, however, were unwilling to give young women a bye. Immersed in a party culture centered on drinking and hooking up, they shrugged off encounters such as Alicia had as unfortunate instances of poor judgment and miscommunication on the part of both partners. Their questions ran along the line of, How's a guy supposed to know that a girl wasn't being coy when she said "No" or "Not right now" or "We should stop"? If a girl regrets what she did the next morning, does that make him a rapist? Sarah, who at twenty-two was one of the older students, summed up their attitudes in an e-mail:

> I feel that it is a woman's responsibility to look after herself and not get into a position where she is uncomfortable or loses control. You can't operate on the assumption that if you want things to stop, the person you are with will respect that. In an ideal world, that would be the case. But we don't live in an ideal world. There are a lot of assholes out there—people who aren't going to care if you change your mind once the clothes have come off. If you make the choice to leave the bar with the guy, then you are also creating the opportunity for something to go wrong—I think that is the point that needs to be driven home to everyone who participates in the hookup culture. Yes, you can practice safe sex. Yes, you can have sex without strings. But this isn't a behavior that doesn't carry risk.

One student told the following story about a friend I'll call Amy.

When Amy arrived at GW as a freshman, she wanted to lose her virginity to someone special. She started hanging out with a guy from her chemistry class and had one of those "in between" relationships so common in the hookup culture—not quite dating, a little more than friends. They would go to parties and kiss on occasion.

One night, her chemistry colleague came over to her dorm room very late and somewhat drunk. He told her he wanted to have sex and brought a bottle of wine to "loosen her up." They drank and started fooling around, but she told him she wasn't ready to have sex.

However, he was. He started by pinning her arms down, ripping off her panties and forcibly inserting his fingers into her, rupturing her hymen as he whispered, "Just relax, and you'll like it." When he began to bite at her neck in drunken lust, she screamed and pushed him off.

"Tease," he said, wiping his bloody hand on the bedsheet before he left.

Amy could not discuss the incident even three years later without trembling.

"It wasn't really assault, because we had been drinking," she said. "And it wasn't rape because we didn't have sex."

Well, then, what was it?

"It was just a bad situation."

Most college codes of conduct, as well as criminal law, would say that what happened to Amy was a crime, not a misfortune. Rape occurs when a person penetrates the anus or vulva of another person without that person's freely given consent. Sexual assault includes rape as well as unwanted sexual touching, again without a stated "Yes" or equally strong signal. The one giving consent must be coherent; if she or he is too drunk to make a choice, consent cannot be assumed.

In Alicia's view, assaults against girls take place because guys don't know how to negotiate what they want, and so resort to demanding or trying it. They also think of themselves in competition with other guys, she says.

"I've had so many guys say you're going to give me blue balls if you don't get me off," she notes. "I wonder what they'd do if I said, 'Go jack off in the bathroom. I mean, it's not pleasant for me to get worked up, either.' "

So why doesn't she say that? For girls like her, as smart and assertive as they appear, the answer has to do at least in part with a poor sense of self-worth, she thinks. "I'm always scared the guy won't like me if I don't give him satisfaction." She may say no once, as she did with both Kevin and Pat, "but they didn't listen and I didn't know how to say it again. My fear of being worthless outweighed my fear of being raped. How messed up is that?"

Duke, like many campuses, offers round-the-clock assistance as part of a comprehensive program to help assault victims. Yet even then, girls like Alicia try to recover on their own—and later find that they haven't. They figure their odds of winning a court conviction are slim, and they're right. According to the U.S. Justice Department, acquaintance rapists are rarely convicted.

"You want justice," psychologist Jean Leonard, Duke's coordinator of sexual assault support services, wrote to Duke students in the spring 2005 edition of a booklet titled *Saturday Night: Untold Stories of Sexual Assault at Duke*.

But what are the odds? You struggle with the rumors that no one has ever been found responsible at Duke (not true), and the belief that large numbers of innocent decent guys are being accused of rape (also not true). And between you and the possibility of justice is the process of recounting every horrible detail of the violation, in front of a board of strangers and the one who harmed you. And the realization that even the "right" decision, the one in your favor, doesn't erase the pain. No matter what, you still have to live with the memory.

Alicia, like Shaida, denied at first the impact the assaults on her had had. She sought out new partners over the rest of her sophomore year. That summer, between sophomore and junior year, she made a visit to

Korea partly in an attempt to find her birth mother, which failed. She hooked up with three guys while she was there.

It was only later that Alicia was able to write to me:

> I can still picture [Kevin's] face and feel his hand over my mouth holding me down into the couch after I told him to stop. I still panic when a guy is on top of me and positions his body so that I feel restricted; even if we are just cuddling or making out. I have punched people when they (innocently) position themselves in the wrong way and I panic and can't get out. This happens even in completely nonsexual situations. I don't think about it every day or when I'm having sex with other people . . . but it's still a memory.

One out of five girls in college will be raped on campus, according to a Justice Department study. Between 85 and 90 percent of the assailants are known by the victim. For some of these young women, life becomes so unbearable that they stop doing their schoolwork, or turn to drugs (particularly cocaine), or attempt suicide, or, like Alicia, quickly start seeking out sex partners again. "They think that this is the way they can prove that the assault didn't affect them," said Catherine Busch, a psychologist who works with victims in suburban Washington, D.C.

TRUST, RESPECT AND OTHER ESSENTIALS

Most young women in high school and college say they want to get married someday. But for people their parents' age and older, it's hard to see how their loosely intimate connections, and the negative attitudes they sometimes adopt as a result of those connections, are preparing them for where they want to end up.

Surprisingly little research has been done on what kinds of relationships lead to good marriages. But the traits that characterize good marriages are firmly established and include trust, respect, admiration, honesty, selflessness, communication, caring and, perhaps more than anything else, commitment. Hookups are about anything but these qualities. It's as if young women are practicing sprints while planning to run a marathon.

Old-fashioned dating had its weaknesses. But it at least forced would-be lovers to think about how they should approach and treat potential partners. If a guy wanted to ask a girl out, he had to give some thought to what she might like to do with him. If he was smart, he also would study her to determine the special qualities she possessed that other guys didn't seem to notice, and remark on them to her. She, thinking, Hey, this guy understands the real me, would agree to go out with him or at least be his friend. For her part she learned that to attract or keep him, she needed to make him feel special by convincing him that he was the only one, or one of very few, who was in her thoughts, her arms or, eventually, her bed.

At first, it could seem like a game. But the more he and she said nice things about each other, the more they came to believe them. With each date they learned more about each other's family, favorite books, political preferences and all the other things that go into making a person unique. They also learned more about themselves. Respect for each other's specialness, as well as respect for themselves, accrued slowly.

The campus lifestyle of young people these days leaves little time to pursue the finer points of a relationship. Even with a serious partner, it's difficult, Alicia said. "At school, you don't do much more than eat together; you're just so busy all day, and when you do try and hang out at night you usually end up passing out from exhaustion. You go out with your own friends and with each other, but only on the weekends, and of course this isn't like 'getting to know you' time really."

Hookup partners spend even less time together. Jumping into bed not only forces decisions they may not be ready to make but kills the chance that they will work at putting their best selves forward. A lot can get lost.

Early one evening in the fall of her junior year, after she returned from Korea, Alicia attended a party with several friends who were seniors and spotted a golden-skinned, handsome guy of average height dancing to a hip-hop tune. He caught her eye and wandered over to talk. She found out that he was a senior and that his name was Chris. Eventually they left the party and walked back to his building. She turned to leave and he asked for her phone number, which she provided.

"He actually called me the next day," she told me a couple of weeks later over coffee, still in shock. "We talked, and he asked if he could call again. On the second or third phone call, he said, 'Every time I talk to you I want to know more about you.' I said to myself, What? Someone wants to get to know me?" In their conversations, she was learning about him, too. She found out he played baseball, occasionally liked to dress in gangsta clothes and was a big fan of the hip-hop singer Talib Kweli.

The first time they dated, Chris picked her up. They had decided in advance to rent a movie and go back to his apartment to watch it. "We talked for, like, three hours," she wrote, "real conversation, not just small talk. We made out for a while, then moved to his bedroom, but before any nakedness happened, I decided to go home. I was proud of myself for not immediately sleeping with him."

They began seeing each other regularly after coming to an understanding about time. As busy as they both were, they would go their separate ways during the week and then spend much of the weekends together. He continued to insist on picking her up at her dorm any time they went out. Such courtesy, commonplace in the 1960s but less so in the decades that followed, astonished Alicia.

"I'd offer to meet him so I wouldn't feel like I owed him anything," she wrote. "But I've been thinking. If we deny chivalry to keep from feeling indebted, but then give ourselves to a guy to keep from feeling guilty, doesn't that just leave us no option but to feel completely used? At least if the guy is being chivalrous, you get some sort of good feelings out of the exchange. Girls should expect that at least."

By the second month of seeing each other, Alicia and Chris realized that they liked each other more than they had anticipated. So they started to talk about breaking up.

They had several reasons. One was the potential for hurt six months hence when Chris was leaving for Japan. Another was the fact that Alicia didn't know if she could trust Chris—or herself, for that matter—to be faithful. "Even if Chris said we should stay together after he graduates, I don't know if I can be alone for a year," she said.

Like Alicia, Chris had had his share of hookups. He had admitted to her before they starting hanging out that he and his roommate had once had a pledge: If they both went out at night, at least one of them had to "get some." She wrote:

> I trust him on some things. I'm getting more comfortable with him emotionally, physically and mentally. But I can't just give up all of me, because I have a core belief that guys are going to hurt me.
>
> When you know someone has hooked up with a lot of people, it's hard to trust them when they do want to commit to you. Bad breakups are enough to harm your ability to trust, but hookups really leave people wary of others.

"Wary" is one adjective that the girls in this book used to describe how hooking up can make them feel about guys, including guys they're interested in. "Cynical" is another, along with "dishonest" and "selfish." Hooking up, as Sienna and Nicole illustrated, is highly adversarial. If you run through lots of casual relationships, seeing your partner as your enemy, the opposite sex can start looking pretty ordinary, or worse. Nicole, who counted up at dinner one night the number of guys she had hooked up with, touched on this when she said, "GW guys are selfish and stupid, the ultimate form of birth control. That's why I only kiss them."

Girls aren't the only ones who can be unkind, as a junior guy at GW demonstrated. This young man kept a condom in his wallet and next to it, a little post-coitus reminder that he had typed and saw every time he reached for a condom.

"Toss the bitches," it read.

Perhaps guys worry that the girls chasing them are taking over yet another role in life that guys used to own. Perhaps they fear that they won't be able to live up to girls' expectations of them in bed. (Campus counselors do, in fact, report an increase in the number of young men complaining of impotence, and the sale of Viagra and other performance-enhancing drugs is brisk among this age group.) Perhaps, even, the guys are afraid of being "tossed" themselves.

With some girls, this may be a legitimate concern. Tonya, a Duke sophomore who went to dinner with me one night along with Shaida and Alicia, talked about enjoying jumping out of bed after having sex, leaving the guy dumbfounded. "To see the look on their face when you get out of bed before they do makes men feel feeble. It gives me such a rush."

Alicia nodded in agreement. "Sometimes you just want to screw them before they screw you." That hardly sounds like practice for a stable relationship.

Suspicion can keep a girl like Victoria away from guys for a whole school year. Or it can persuade a girl like Cleo to stay with a guy like Steven, even when she isn't in love with him, because she fears anyone else would be a creep.

Of course, Cleo cheated on Steven. When hooking up becomes a habit, it's hard to break. Jessica, a junior, brought this up in my class at

GW, admitting that she was beginning to get bored sexually in her eight-month relationship. "I really prefer sex when I'm in a relationship," she said. "But I lose interest quickly. I like the thrill of a new sexual encounter."

Sarah, a graduate student, knew what her classmate was talking about. She, too, had been in semi-serious relationships where "you still act like you're on the hunt, even though you don't need to be."

This led a third student, Brian, to ask, "Is the monogamous marriage a thing of the past?"

Some college students who hook up argue that they'll be less likely to cheat once they're in a committed relationship. Cheating frequently comes from wanting something other than what you have, they say. If they sample a number of possible partners before deciding what they want, they'll be less likely to be unfaithful when they do settle down. This was the position Alicia and Chris had taken separately before they met. But once they had reached the two-month mark, they realized it wasn't easy to get beyond their past. They wanted to talk honestly about former liaisons but had difficulty doing that. Hooking up, with its ambiguities and innuendos, had given them little practice in straight talk or negotiating different points of view.

Robert Blum, a physician and professor of psychology at Johns Hopkins University, worries about the lessons that go unlearned in today's casually sexual culture. "In traditional boyfriend-girlfriend relationships," he says, "you begin to understand how someone else thinks about things. You learn the skill of compromise, and not to say the first thing on your mind. You learn how to say you're sorry and accept other people's apologies." These fundamental skills for both private and public life can also be learned from parents and platonic friends. But, in his view, they may be best learned within a romantic relationship because the young person is motivated by the *romance* to learn them.

Lloyd Kolbe, the health education professor at Indiana University, is particularly troubled by the absence in hooking up of an ethic of caring. Children and adolescents learn to care for others, and what it's like to be cared for, in their interactions with parents, close friends and romantic partners, he says. He still remembers his first love in high school, how he worked at being honest, decent and caring—in short, worthy of her.

"Hooking up is purposely uncaring," he says. "If they turn off the emotional spigot during this time, what will happen to them as older adults?

"Perhaps there's nothing wrong with casual sexual relationships among unmarried, uncommitted people, both of whom have the same expectations," he concedes. "We don't have any data supporting the idea that psychological problems result from early intercourse in and of itself."

But eventually, he says, "if we're treated in an uncaring way by others over and over again, we will likely respond in kind. The effect down the road could be exponential."

ISO: GREAT SEX

Hooking up may be all about sex—the use of sex to land a guy or the pursuit of a guy to get sex. But it's not about good sex, let alone great sex. It's not about the kind that can emerge after the first wave of lust, when caring about and trusting someone allows each partner to experiment with what gives them the most pleasure. It's not about the sex that puts a spring in your step and makes you carry yourself with self-confidence. The girls I observed almost always ended up disappointed by sex.

Remember Mieka, the high school junior who read a magazine while her partner had sex with her? She wasn't the only girl I interviewed who admitting to "checking out" while her guy got off.

"Hookups are very scripted," Alicia said. "You're supposed to know what to do and how to do it and how to feel during and afterward. You learn to turn everything off except your body and make yourself emotionally invulnerable."

In other words, you make yourself passionless. Hooking up may not risk the emotional lows of a failed relationship, but its highs are not nearly as high as what you can feel if you're in love—with or without sex toys.

"From the time I lost my virginity until now (with Chris)," Alicia said, "it's only been the guy getting pleasure. After I had sex the first time, it became much less of a big deal. I could take it almost as casually as making out, as long as I didn't feel threatened. . . . More guys have had sex with me than I have had sex with them. I guess this is the kind of sex where the guy is just using my vagina to get himself off. The best part of being on bottom in these hookups is you don't have to do any work."

More than a century ago, a young man could bring a blush to a young woman's cheeks by holding her hand or her eyes a bit too long. A young woman could excite a young man merely by picking up her gown ever so slightly, revealing a finely turned ankle. Similar flirtations play out today. But after they've been acknowledged, the race toward having sex is on.

In the past, partners took time between steps and, as they did, learned about the other person, increasing both the anticipation and the pleasure. Kissing was an initial goal, then lost some of its allure and was replaced by petting, which was replaced by intercourse, and sometimes by oral and anal sex as well. It's one thing to become careless about one or two avenues to pleasure, but is this generation, or the one that will come after it, on its way to being indifferent to all of them? Have the joys of sit-down dinners been replaced by a regular diet of Big Macs at the drive-thru?

Listen to Alicia wax wistful about the old days:

These days holding hands in public has more significance than having sex. I was thinking about how easily people will go to bed with
someone, but how freaked out they would be if they had to walk
around sober holding that person's hand. Sex used to be something
that was intimate, and now it can almost impede intimacy in the traditional romantic sense. I realized the other day how long it's been
since I've had a boyfriend I would walk around holding hands with.
I miss that life.

Now listen to her describe a night during her summer visit to Korea.
She had met a guy named Chae at a club, dined with him and accompanied him to his apartment.

We had sex. I was too tired to give him head, feeling guilty about not
getting him off somehow and too tired to think up an excuse not to
have sex, so I just let him do it. This happens in more situations than
I like, where I say you can use my body but I'm not doing anything
to help you. . . . He left for America a little bit later, but we are still
in touch. . . . I don't feel anything for him friend- or relationship-wise.

When she returned home late that summer, she resumed hooking up
regularly with a guy she had started to see before she went overseas.

I hated sleeping with [Dan]. First, he just assumed we would have sex.
He would look at me with an expectant face when he wasn't hard
enough and tell me to "suck it." It took him forever, and it wasn't en-
joyable for me. He had a bit of a beer gut, which I think is the most
unattractive thing ever, and he sweated a lot. But then again, outside
of bed, he was a good guy. We had a lot of great conversations. . . .
It was certainly not the time for a relationship, and I think we both

knew that. At the time, I felt like I would see him again, and now I could care less.

Given the clinical way in which sex is described in most classrooms, it's not surprising that many young people are so matter-of-fact about having sex and bewildered when feelings intervene. Since the late 1970s and the AIDS scare, sex-education classes have focused almost completely on the physical: body parts, pregnancy and health risks. Recently, the federal government's drive to force abstinence-only curricula into the schools has limited the ability of public-school teachers even more to engage their students in any kind of discussion about sex, including sex and love.

A Manhattan professional in her mid-twenties offered another explanation for this ho-hum attitude. After a series of flings, she told me, "Instead of sitting at home crying because John didn't call us, we force ourselves to think we didn't care if he called anyway. Does that part of us that seeks connection eventually start to break down when we no longer associate sex with love?"

Of course, fireworks do not always accompany sex in an exclusive relationship, either. Physical urges come and go, the machinery may not always hum and stress or fatigue will certainly interfere. The point is, such failings kill hookups but usually do not threaten committed relationships.

Good relationships, like good marriages, are about commitment, perhaps more than anything else. Love is wonderful, but it's also fickle, and one can fall out of love. Respect, trust and caring are crucial, but on occasion even the most loving partner will have a bad day and take it out on the person closest to him or her. Commitment forgives, or at least outlives. College women say they're not ready to commit, and indeed many may not be. But that doesn't mean they don't think about it.

It's little wonder they shy away from it: Older adults make commitment seem about as desirable as signing your life away to the Army because it beats being the greeter at Wal-Mart. Young adults know they don't want to be single all their lives but have few models of what they'd like to be or how to get there. These young people have grown up in a country where almost one out of two marriages end in divorce and divorced partners frequently go on to marry and divorce again. The United States has the highest rate of transitional living arrangements of any Western nation, with four times as many American children living in three or more parental partnerships as children in Sweden. One result of such dislocations can be seen in the attitudes of children from divorced families, the majority of whom, when asked about marriage, say it's forever "if things work out." Fewer than one out of two children from intact families say the same thing.

Alicia, who admired her parents' marriage, said the larger culture had influenced her. She wrote, "We never see anything positive about Hollywood relationships. It's beginning to seem normal to get married on flings and then get divorced and have random babies. . . . I guess that's how the media get you. They don't directly change your opinions, but over time you begin to feel like everyone is doing it."

She concluded, "I think our generation is less likely to stick around and work out problems in a marriage."

Commitment is something grander than sticking around to work out problems. It is saying to your partner that he is your number one priority, not necessarily the person who provides the best sex or is the smartest or wealthiest or most fun to be with. Like a parent to a child, you're dedicated to the relationship, not just to the person, to making it work despite obstacles. You're also willing to sacrifice some of your preferences for the good of the relationship. Your partner is saying the same thing to you, and for both of you the relationship is not so much a contract you can't escape but a team you won't quit—except under unusual circumstances. You come to appreciate each other's differences and learn from them, expanding who you are in a way you could not have done alone.

Alicia began to realize what she and Chris contributed to each other after winter break. He, majoring in international studies and French, was creative and chafed under structured school assignments. She, the engineer, helped him figure out when the rules were necessary while he encouraged her to look at her work from a variety of perspectives. She admired how close he was to his parents but encouraged him to make more decisions without their input. He told her he admired her independence but suggested she work to improve relationships at home. They both started studying each other more intentionally and talking more often about what they observed. "We both feel better together than apart," she said.

According to Alicia, they did these things after they had asked each other, "Are we just friends who hook up or do we have obligations to each other?" Their conversations were difficult, coming as they did out of a past of mostly hookups. But they decided that they had "a commitment to be in this relationship," even if it didn't last forever. They left themselves an escape: "We won't draw this out past the time when it is no longer a mutual choice."

Laurence Steinberg, the psychology professor at Temple, suggests that most college graduates become serious about pairing up in their middle to late twenties and then start the rehearsals that will prepare them in their thirties for marriage. He suggests that all they're doing at the moment is continuing a trend toward later first marriages that began more than two decades ago. He also notes that the divorce rate is lower among women who married at age twenty-five and older, so a reluctance to tie the knot is not necessarily a bad thing.

Robert Blum, at Johns Hopkins, agrees that for these middle- and upper-income young people, hooking up may be just a holding pattern. But he worries about the effects of a shortened timetable once they decide to settle down.

"It's one thing to say relationships can wait when you're twelve," he says. "It's something else to say 'I'll wait until I'm thirty to get my personal life in order.' If you do not have experience with forming relationships earlier, your likelihood of entering into a relationship later that can be sustained over time is at risk. It's like taking an exam assuming you'll do well without experience in the subject, lots of studying and lots of practice."

Once young people graduate from college, they don't necessarily start dating successfully. Far from it. Online dating services wouldn't be pulling in millions of dollars if young adults knew how to date on their own. Fashion and makeup consultants wouldn't be able to charge $350 or more an hour to prepare a woman for a date. Books like *The Rules*, promising to show young women how to capture the man of their dreams, wouldn't become best sellers. And let's not forget that a large number of twentysomethings are not all that eager to date. One national survey of eighteen- to twenty-nine-year-olds reported that almost 60 percent were not in committed relationships, and the majority were not interested in being in one. When the survey was released, I interviewed a dozen twentysomethings. The reaction of a twenty-six-year-old assistant at a Manhattan talent agency was typical. "A relationship takes so much time and energy," she said, "and there's so much stuff I want to do with my career. I'm not that interested in looking."

Here's something else to think about: When girls do decide they're ready to mate, whether that's at twenty-five, thirty or later, will guys be ready? Or have they had it so good for so long that they see no reason to settle down?

As people get older and marry, the possible pool of partners contracts, Blum notes. Young women may end up choosing a mate they might not otherwise have selected. Their ability to have children shrinks as well. "If you say I'm going to put off forming relationships until I'm thirty, you have a very small window to be successful."

CHILDREN, FULL-TIME

In the last part of the nineteenth century, nearly one-half of the women who graduated from college remained unmarried and childless. "They could marry or they could become 'professionals'—teachers, librarians, social workers," Gail Collins writes in her book *America's Women*. "Almost no one felt they could do both. Even union leaders and college presidents retired when they became wives. Frequently, educated women opted for jobs over husbands."

Today, a young educated woman can also enjoy a full life without a ring on her left hand or a baby carriage beside her. Just as working as a consultant, rather than for one company, satisfies some people, composing a personal life of serial good times with interesting people may be a fine way to live.

Beginning in the 1960s, the number of Americans choosing to remain unmarried began to climb. By the year 2000, these solos made up 31.6 percent of all homes, a slightly higher proportion than couples with children, married and unmarried combined. Trend watchers now talk about "tribes" of single people replacing married couples in the suburbs, and people like Thomas Coleman, who runs an association called Unmarried America, suggest that women are part of this trend. Their self-esteem, he says, "isn't based on having children and being married anymore."

But for young women who want to have children—and the vast majority say they do—there are certain job requirements. The evidence is pretty clear that, all other factors being equal, children do best being raised by two competent, caring parents (including stepparents) who are committed to each other and to the children. Single parents can excel at being moms and dads, although their job is harder, and they, too, must be able to put their children first for twenty-one years. With kids you can't be a temp, walking away at the first sign of trouble or if you get a better job offer. Your home is not a hotel.

If hooking up, which is by definition self-centered and selfish, becomes a way of thinking about, and acting in, relationships, it is fair to ask what impact that might have on efforts to build and support a family. Women already are signaling that they feel they don't need to be married to be mothers. In 2004, half of births to women in their early twenties and nearly three in ten births to women twenty-five to twenty-nine were to unmarried women, up considerably from previous years. Presumably most of these women were in some kind of relationship, but we don't know for how long.

Anecdotally, I can't count how many young women have told me that if they don't meet the right man by their early to middle thirties, they'll either adopt or make a trip to the sperm bank and pursue motherhood on their own. Shaida, for one, told me she dreamed of raising a child without a spouse. If she follows through on that, will she be able to handle her son's or daughter's inevitable crankiness, stubbornness, illness and other problems with patience and good sense? If she finds a partner, will she be able to work through their inevitable differences over the best way to raise a child? Will her partner? The odds are that he, too, will have had little practice at being a partner or a father.

Alicia knew she wanted to be a mother. Because she does not know her birth parents, her children would be her first blood kin, she said. She spoke with pride about the relationship she had seen between her adoptive parents, which she called "cutely affectionate." Her mother and father read the Bible together, she said, frequently asking their children to join them. While she did not share their religious beliefs, she appreciated the time they spent with each other and the rest of the family.

Her desire for family was not always applauded: As a senior in high school, she was cut from a scholarship competition after she told the panel interviewing her that her number one goal in life was to raise a family. "Apparently," she said later, "they wanted something more along the lines of developing innovative technology to save the world." She couldn't see why eventually she couldn't do both.

CONNECTING TO WORK

The parallel between hookup relationships and this generation's work habits is striking. Marisa Nightingale, senior director of media programs for the National Campaign to Prevent Teen Pregnancy, was one of the first to point this out to me. She was in a good position to comment because she listens to older teens talk about sexuality and relationships and also regularly hires young people in their twenties, mostly females, for positions with the campaign. In her early thirties, she is not that many years older than those she hires and is a popular boss.

Her employees, she said, "are highly individualistic, very mobile workers. They never stay in one place very long." The day of our interview she had finished looking over dozens of applications for the position of her assistant. "More than fifty percent of them were in their late twenties and had never worked in one place longer than a year. If work got too hard or too boring or too tedious, they'd leave—just like in their relationships."

Others confirm her impression about this generation's work habits. "They are well aware of the fact that they will not work for the same company for the rest of their life," says Bill Frey, a demographer with the Brookings Institution, a think tank in Washington. "They don't think long term about health care or Social Security. They're concerned about their careers and immediate gratification." He points out that companies, for their part, aren't necessarily looking for permanent relationships with employees, either, partly because short-term relationships tend to be cheaper.

"We want everything right away," Alicia says. "It's our MO, the way we think about technology, cars, everything, including relationships."

Certainly these young women won't need all the same attributes required of previous generations of workers. But won't they need skills in communication? Or problem-solving? Or teamwork? Or other traits one learns in a relationship?

Earlier in this book, I argued that the fact that young women expect to move around in their twenties, working in various jobs, traveling if they can afford it, serving in the Peace Corps or similar agencies, makes hookups and other short-term relationships more appealing than serious connections. Could the influence also run in the other direction? Could hooking up feed certain attitudes that extend into careers? Will they say, "I'm going to work everything to my advantage rather than put someone else's welfare ahead of my own"? Or, "If I wade into a project at work that is more difficult than I expected, or that I don't like, I'll try to find a way to shift it off onto someone else. If that doesn't work, maybe I'll take a hike"?

THE END AND A BEGINNING

By late spring of our year together, secure in her feelings for Chris and with her bouts of depression and anorexia mostly behind her, Alicia was moving ahead at top speed. She was chosen to lead a team of engineering students to Indonesia in August to repair shrimp hatcheries damaged by the 2004 tsunami. She applied for and was accepted into a program in Barcelona in early summer that would enable her to obtain a certificate for teaching English overseas. She started fielding inquiries from engineering firms about jobs after graduation even though it was a year away. She wrote papers and studied for finals in her five courses—three in engineering, one in psychology and one in sociology—and made straight A's, her best grades ever. As sorority social chair, she continued to throw great parties.

She also started saying goodbye to Chris, who was on his way overseas. He told her that given their ambitious and uncertain plans, they shouldn't commit themselves to a future together yet. She agreed. She needed to be single again. At this stage in their lives, a good relationship did not have to last forever.

They talked about meeting in Paris during the summer. On the day he left campus, she wrote to me:

> It's hard to know that being apart is what has to happen. For someone who has held me as we sleep and been there when I wake up, for someone whom I have shared all my highs and lows with, it is a hard goodbye. But Chris is right. Neither of us is ready to be in something so serious yet. There is too much left to develop within us as individuals. We will be, as he puts it, "sexier" the next time we see each other.

They met in Paris in mid-July and spent five days walking around the city, kissing, arguing, kissing, trading insults and kissing some more. In Montmartre, Chris asked a sidewalk artist to paint Alicia's portrait. They climbed the Eiffel Tower.

As they stood three hundred meters high looking over the City of Light, Chris asked, "What would you do if I proposed to you right now?"

She didn't hesitate.

"I'd like you to propose on top of a building *I* built."

Later she told me, "We kissed a lot that day. But what meant the most to me was that he was standing there with me at the top of the tower and seeing what I was seeing, understanding what I was understanding." It was the last time she saw him before returning to Duke for her senior year. It also happened to be Bastille Day—commemorating the day in 1789 when the French people proclaimed independence.

For all of their eight months together, they had known this day would come. Unlike many of their friends, they had said yes to building a relationship anyway as long as they could make it work. In her mind it had been, to take the title of one of her term papers, "a beautiful struggle." She was proud of them both.

My generation—actually our society—is into taking shortcuts. . . . Get rich faster. Skip this step. Win instant approval. Hookups are like the shortcut to intimacy, while dating is the long way around, the scenic route. We want to get there, wherever "there" is, as quickly as possible, and I think we've lost the ability to enjoy the journey.

Sometimes we forget that how much the "end" means depends on the "means" you took to get there. Sometimes patience is a virtue. I think some people are starting to realize that the intimacy learned from a hookup is no match for the intimacy from a relationship. However, they aren't quite sure what the difference is. They don't recognize that the process of dating/getting to know someone/caring for someone is very important in creating the depth of feeling you will have for them. Or that you don't have to marry someone in order to learn from spending time with them. There are some relationships that aren't going anywhere, but you can still learn about yourself, even if it's only to stand up and tell the guy he's not what you need.

Neither Alicia nor any of the other girls I interviewed believe that dating will return to campuses anytime soon. In an e-mail at the end of the year, Alicia told me why, unwittingly summing up much of what I had seen at her campus and others.

For one thing, you have the whole movement to make college campuses self-sustaining. Your food, dorm, sports, entertainment are all right on campus, and this doesn't exactly encourage dating. Two, you have the peer pressure and societal pressure to move through things quickly, to not get tied down, to be an independent woman to the exclusion of boyfriends. Three, dating is a drain on energy and intellect, and we are overworked, overprogrammed and overcommitted just trying to get to grad school, let alone marriage. I think it's rare to find someone who would want to put their relationships over their academics/future. I don't even know that relationships are seen as an integrated part of this whole "future" idea. Sometimes I think they are on their own track that runs parallel and that we feel can be pushed aside or drawn closer at our whim. And last is the distance/time thing. We are a mobile culture, and we're not supposed to settle down until thirtyish.

She had one thought: Maybe if girls invested more of themselves in improving the connections to people already in their lives—including their parents and friends of both genders—the depth of romantic encounters would improve as well. She wrote me:

Right now in college, love is seen as a game of luck. We wander around meeting tons of people, each with our own personal arsenal of huge life plans, and we make new friends and hook up with people and collide in many different ways. It is just luck if you happen upon that guy whom you happen to click with. Perhaps an idea is to turn this game of luck into a game of skill . . . the skill of developing meaningful relationships.

And what role should sex play in that game?

"The dating culture assumed women own sex and men have to work to get it," she wrote. "The hookup culture assumes women own sex and have to give it up. Maybe sex is owned by both partners and should be pursued by mutual agreement."

CODA

Almost a year to the day that I lectured at Duke about hooking up, and listened later to Jamie's grievances about her experiences during her freshman year, I returned to the same classroom to lead a similar discussion with a fresh batch of public-policy students.

Our conversation was much the same as the one twelve months earlier: energetic, direct and highly ambivalent about relationships on campus. If anything, this class was more critical of hooking up than the previous one. This time, as students volunteered what they liked and didn't like about hooking up, I asked the teaching assistant to keep count on the blackboard in front of us. Four positives emerged ("You're free to try out different guys and girls" was one) and twelve negatives ("Makes you cynical").

Were they giving me the answers they thought I wanted to hear? Or expressing how they really felt? I believe it was some of both. These were smart kids, their generation by many accounts more practical than my generation. But the chaos of hooking up was getting to them, just as it had to Jamie and the other girls in this book.

As the bell rang and the class departed, a student approached me just as Jamie had the year before. Like Jamie, this student was in a long-distance relationship. The hookup culture was making them question their commitment, the student said, and they had broken up three times so far. Should they abandon each other and hook up? Or keep trying to stay together? Did I have any advice at all?

This time, the student was a fraternity guy in T-shirt, cargo shorts and cap.

Although they don't admit it readily, young men are as dissatisfied with hooking up as young women. If the culture is going to change, it will take both to change it. That won't happen, however, until they have opportunities to think about it smartly and ask each other questions such as: What about hooking up do they want to preserve? What do they want to toss? Are there characteristics of old-fashioned dating that they would like to restore? What would a new model of relating look like?

Well before kids go to college, parents can prepare them for this kind of introspection by insisting that they have some downtime each week, and that they make decisions on their own that get increasingly tougher with each year. A sense of personal competence is key. Parents also can demonstrate that two people in a long-term relationship may actually enjoy each other's company by going on dates and, like Victoria's mother and father, being openly affectionate with each other.

But parents need not be the only teachers or, as their kids get older, discussion leaders. Schools could play a significant role. Right now, educators are largely divided between conservatives who think teachers should never talk about sex in the classroom except to say "Wait until you're married," and liberals who focus on sex and protecting one's body. Either approach, by itself, is doomed to fail because each ignores the way girls and guys actually live their lives. What is needed is some movement toward the "radical middle": education that is comprehensive and draws on young people's day-to-day experiences.

Apart from this book, there is abundant evidence that young people are hungry for this kind of information and discussion. Cathy Small, an anthropology professor at Northern Arizona University, spent a year undercover as a freshman at a large university, taking classes, eating meals and sleeping in a dorm. In her book *My Freshman Year*, which she wrote under a pseudonym, she recounts having many late-night conversations with young women in the dorm where she stayed, and each night before she went to bed, she tabulated the subjects of each discussion. Eighty-eight topics were covered, and a third of them involved what she called "boys, meeting boys and sex." Those subjects were by far the most popular, she said.

Robin Sawyer, a public-health professor, has been teaching his course in human sexuality at the University of Maryland for twenty years. The course includes the psychological and social aspects of sexuality. It is so popular that he has to cap it at 250 students every semester, and confine the class mostly to seniors. This, as he notes, is a pity, since it is precisely the kind of course freshmen need in order to prepare them for what they'll find on campus.

His students, and millions of others, are more than capable of reflecting on and refining the way they spend their intimate moments. The question is whether they should have to do so among themselves, alone.

A Letter to Mothers
and Daughters

I f you are a woman who came of age during the women's movement of the 1960s and 1970s, I suspect you believe, as I do, that we have a responsibility to reach out and help other women improve their lives. This means especially the next generation: our daughters all, moving through adolescence into young adulthood.

We have not been shy about advising them on matters of the mind: their schoolwork, careers and checking accounts. We have attempted to do our duty on matters of the body as well, including how to avoid pregnancy, unwanted babies and sexually transmitted infections. Some of us have even attempted, largely unsuccessfully, to suggest how they should dress. It is now time—past time, in fact—to widen our lens, to start a new dialogue with them on matters that connect the mind, body and heart.

I have engaged young women in such discussions for almost a decade. Of late I have been nagged by a question: Do I have an obligation not only to provide a faithful description of what they say and do, but also to give them the best advice I can offer? From what I've seen and heard, particularly in researching this book, our daughters are hungry for conversations with older women about sex, love and the relationship between the two. They may not start such discussions, but if we do, they will, in time, jump in if they feel we are listeners, not judges.

They will, and should, make up their own minds. But they also want to know what we think. Our job is to give them something to think about. We can't change what they see, but we can help them change the way they see it.

We have resisted this. Some of us, when we were their age, rebelled against the sexual rules of our time and are not sure what to pass on. Some of us made mistakes when choosing romantic partners and feel we have no authority to speak about such matters. Many of us feel that their social world is so different from the one we grew up in that anything we say would be worthless.

These are legitimate concerns, but they're not legitimate reasons for keeping silent. Young people need to hear what we consider the essentials of loving relationships, as half-thought-out as our ideas may be. They need to hear about our failed attempts at intimacy so that when they fail, they won't be afraid to try again.

The curfews and other conventions that we both resisted and relied upon are gone, and much of that is our doing. We questioned the social structures that reinforced sexual double standards and were right to do so. But we put nothing in their place, and without them, today's young women are having to write their own rules, which is a much harder task than we ever faced. We must let them know that they do not have to do it alone.

For the purposes of this letter, I have chosen as my daughters the young women in the book. I urge you, as women, to start a conversation with your daughters, whoever they might be.

Dear Daughters,

You are not mine. You were not mine to raise, torture or love. But over our time together—our hours upon hours of interviews, lunches, dinners, parties, shopping expeditions and e-mail exchanges—I have come to care for you as if you were my own. We have examined the tenderest spots of your strong yet tender souls, and both you and I have been changed.

They say that parents grow up with their children. I feel that way about you. Observing your life and loves has forced me to think about my life and loves, and I thank you for that opportunity.

By way of goodbye, allow me to give you some parting advice, worded more straightforwardly than I previously talked to you. Some of these thoughts are mine alone, but most of them reflect what you have taught me about how you wish to relate to intimate others, even if your daily behaviors occasionally suggested otherwise.

LOVING YOURSELF

♦ *A guy can make you feel valuable, but it's not the guy who makes you valuable.*

You are the subject of your life, not someone else's life: not your parents', your friends' or your partner's. On the outside you may look like you could take on the world. But you and I know that on many days you feel pretty ordinary, and that's when you're vulnerable to doing things that whittle away at your self-confidence.

It's okay to feel ordinary right now. You're still figuring you out—your purpose, your principles, what and who will help you get where you want to go. Take advantage of the choices you have that build inner confidence, and not just the choices in the college catalogue. Learn to scuba dive. Teach a child to read. Invest in good friendships. Explore intimacy within relationships. Avoid hookups. They'll make you feel more ordinary than you already feel—and look more ordinary to the guy you set your sights on. He will seek to win you over only if he thinks you're a prize.

The more confident you become, independent of love, the more confident you will be in love.

Consider your life to come. Years from now, do you really want to recall banging bodies with a partner in bed while your roommate was typing her political science paper nearby? Do you want to risk being invited to a dinner party and realize once you get there that you have hooked up with every guy in the room? How will you feel on your first or second job when a colleague mentions seeing a webcam photo of you and a former partner in the nude?

Career counselors have told you that thinking about what kind of job you eventually want will help you decide how to prepare. This holds true for the personal as well. In ten or fifteen years, do you want to be living with a husband or a long-term partner? Raising kids? Both? Are your sexual and romantic encounters teaching you the skills you'll need to find and sustain what you desire?

◆ *Don't let them have what you've got until you, and they, know who you are.*

Your body is your property. No one has a right to enter unless you welcome them in. Think about the first home you hope to own. You wouldn't want someone to throw a rock through the front window, would you? Is your body worth less than a house?

Think of it this way: Your body is not an introductory offer. It's a return receipt. Your partner gives you love or at least respect and affection, and in return you give him part of you—and you decide which part.

Respecting yourself means also respecting the person you've chosen to be with. So when you say "I'm worth waiting for," you should also be saying "And so are you." If your partner is not worth waiting for, he or she is not worth it, period.

♦ *Explore your feminine side beyond the black lace bra.*

Would you like a guy to open the door for you or invite you to dinner? Seek out someone who will do that. Experience how it feels to tell your girlfriends "He is taking me out" as opposed to "We are going out." Ask him how he feels playing the gallant and show him how much you appreciate it by offering a genuine "Thank you" in return. You don't need to do anything else. You're doing him a favor by allowing him to show you his best manners.

Extend special courtesies to the person you're interested in as well. Open the door for him when his arms are full of books, and take him out to dinner when he's feeling blue. Neither of you should get hung up on gender stereotypes when it comes to making the other feel special.

♦ *Admit it, the bar scene is a guy thing.*

Tying one on can be fun occasionally. Just don't let it take over your social life. Organize weekend getaways and other events to bring people together. Bake cookies, brownies, muffins. Ask your girlfriends for assistance. Guys will do anything for homemade baked goods.

LOVING ANOTHER WELL

♦ *Love won't change you; it will just make you more of who you are.*

Do not be afraid of your need to love. It is hardwired, improving our species' chance for survival. Loving another makes you more giving, more relaxed and more adventurous. In a good relationship, you like who you both are when you're together—and who you are both becoming.

You delight in finding out that he hates frogs, and he relishes knowing your secret love of NASCAR. He makes your A in chemistry seem amazing, and you convince him his C in sociology is a onetime aberration. You hated bowling in high school, but he likes it, so you agree to give it another try. With him your joy is amplified and your sadness lessened. Yes, you can be sad in front of him. You can also be confused and upset. If he loves you, he will love your vulnerabilities as well as your strengths.

◆ *Lust is not love, although it can feel like it.*

Is sex what you want? Or is it a means to a relationship? If the latter, rethink the order of things. Anyone can get laid, but only a few will get laid and loved the first time. A loving relationship is much more likely to happen *before* you hook up than afterward.

◆ *Do you want to be the love of someone's life or live with someone who's the love of your life?*

There are two kinds of men: those who make you feel comfortable and secure, and those who keep you living on the edge of passion—and doubt.

With whom are you happiest? And with whom will you be happiest ten years from now? The answers may not be the same. Just remember: Sexual attraction, though wonderful and essential, waxes and wanes. Our need for companionship is constant. Maybe you'll get lucky and find one man who is both. In case you don't, these questions are worth considering.

◆ *The past is prologue.*

Remember your first love? Of course you do. What did you get from that relationship that you want to find again? What do you want to avoid?

Think of other relationships and hookups. Which memories pop up first? The time that guy peeled an orange for you as you lay sick in bed with the flu? Or the guy in the bar who kept buying you shots with the promise that he'd take you—where was it again? Home?

In his poem "This Much I Do Remember," Billy Collins calls these recollections "coins of the moment." He writes:

Even after I have forgotten what year it is,
my middle name,
and the meaning of money,
I will still carry in my pocket
the small coin of the moment,
minted in the kingdom
that we pace through every day.

You're filling up your purse with coins every day. When you open it several years from now, what will you find? What would you like to find?

◆ *Breaking up* is *hard to do—and instructive.*

Falling in love is easy; staying in love is work. Life gets in the way. If you want to keep working at a relationship, that's love. If you must call it quits, don't beat yourself up about it. People fail at love all the time. They also start over.

Whether your relationship dissolves or a hookup leaves you sour, you will discover some of the same lessons. You need space and time to discern them. Take a sabbatical. Otherwise you risk making the same mistakes again.

◆ *Even with a good guy, you'll still need friends.*

Relying on a boyfriend to provide the essentials of friendship is not only unrealistic but also dangerous. An otherwise lovely relationship can collapse under such expectations.

You need the friendship of other young women, and you'll find out who your true pals are once you get involved with a guy. A real friend will take pleasure in your pleasure, not be jealous or find a way to belittle your joy. She'll be the first to cry foul if you've been hooking up with a guy for a month and he keeps saying he doesn't want to "date" you. She'll also tell you when you're being a jerk.

Discover the joy of friendships with women older than you. Press these women on questions such as: Which of the old ways of dating are worth saving, and which would they ditch if they were you? Talk to them about what you expect from guys, what you hope for, what you've gotten so far and what you're afraid of.

Finding someone older whom you're comfortable with may not be easy, but she is out there. She may be a wise aunt, the mother of your best friend, a favorite professor. Consider talking to a female pastor or rabbi. Her sense of a purposeful life and a deep faith, rooted in history, may help ground you.

GOOD SEX, BAD SEX

◆ *Think erotic, not pornographic.*

Pornographic is grinding on the dance floor like a dog in heat. It leaves nothing to the imagination. Erotic is a meticulously calculated promise of something that may or may not happen: a lingering gaze, a sultry smile, a silk blouse unbuttoned one button too many or a long lick of an ice cream cone.

A hookup can be convenient. It requires no maintenance. Your partner's little quirks don't annoy you because you know you won't be around for long. You make no attempt to change each other's lives. In your head, he can be anything you want him to be.

But be honest, it's not erotic. There's no savoring the ride; the ride is over before you know it. Hooking up is like taking the final plunge down a giant roller coaster without first experiencing the nail-biting anticipation of the climb to the top. It's a cheap thrill that's not all that thrilling.

◆ *Sex always has meaning, even when it is "meaningless."*

Sex can be abusive and selfish, or it can reinforce our best qualities: our playfulness, generosity, sense of responsibility and trustworthiness.

Be honest with yourself about every sexual act in which you engage. Do you like what you're doing? Does it feel not only good but right? What is your inner voice telling you? "Full speed ahead"? "Slow down"? "Stop"? If you're moving toward intercourse during a hookup, first ask yourself, "Do I really want to do this?" not "Is he wearing a condom?" (That comes second.)

Sex alone won't make him yours. You may feel close immediately after you hook up, but that's simply your body's chemicals kicking in. His body doesn't react the same way, and he may well start thinking of you as a hookup partner rather than someone to love.

Let's say you're both drunk. To whom are you and he making love? If it takes liquor to feel a connection to someone, the connection isn't there. Work on it when you're sober.

Don't have sex because he wants you to or you think it will make you feel special. It won't. If you don't believe this, wait until he has sex with someone else and see how special you feel. Or find out who else he has hooked up with. That's the "special" group you're about to join.

The bottom line is that hookups aren't meant to be special. In a smorgasbord of booty, all the hot dishes start looking like they've been on the warming table too long.

USING POWER WISELY
◆ *Plan your dive and dive your plan.*

This is the first rule for scuba divers, and it applies in social encoun-

ters as well. You're going to find yourself in situations where you wonder, "Should I say yes to this?" "How about now?" "Is this still okay?"
If you have a plan, you'll be more likely to arrive at the right answer.

You possess a lot more power before you sleep with a guy than afterward. Think more about when to say "Yes" than when to say "No."
Even if you've said yes before, you can say no the next time. Why not
rethink it every time and at every stage?

If you make the first move, do it deliberately, with forethought. Think
about how much of yourself you're willing to give the first or second
time you're with him.

There's one exception to the plan rule: The most memorable kisses
are frequently the ones you don't anticipate.

P.S. Don't flirt with a guy if you're not interested in him. That will
only hurt and confuse him and encourage him to mistreat girls.

◆ *The personal is the political.*

You do not have to choose the dating options presented to you. You
can come up with your own. But you cannot follow through alone. You
will need the support of girlfriends who also want to change things. Forget competing with girls for the title of prettiest or skinniest or the one
who has the highest number of hookups. That's so middle school.

If individuals consider hooking up only in terms of what it does for
or to them, nothing will change. So tell people when you said no to a guy.
Support other girls who walk away from situations that made them un-
easy. Assist girls who didn't walk away and feel they made a mistake. Talk
over alternatives.

◆ *You're in this together.*

The hookup culture is regrettably adversarial, pitting girls against
guys. Don't buy into its cynicism. As much as they may act like it some-

times, guys are not the enemy. Don't excuse their bad behavior, but do try to understand it.

Guys are frequently intimidated by girls who seem to be able to do everything well. Sexually aggressive girls in particular scare them. What if they aren't super-studs in bed? they wonder. What if that got out among their guy friends? Better to take a girl by force, some of them think, than have their masculinity questioned.

They're not going to slow things down on their own. They've grown up in a cut-to-the-chase popular culture of action/adventure flicks and fast-paced video games and have little patience for leisurely plots. Besides, hooking up is ideal for them: It is simple and doesn't require a lot of preparation, reading of signals or attention to feelings.

Eventually, many guys find hooking up unsatisfying, too. But it takes them longer to recognize and verbalize their discomfort. Girls must bring them along in their thinking.

So insist on talking about what you both are considering doing. Say what you would like to do and what you won't do. Ask them to do the same. Guys are more literal-minded than girls; try not to hear more than what they said. Clarify if you're unsure.

You are ultimately in this together because when the playing field is leveled, either everyone wins or everyone loses.

One final note: Share these thoughts with other girls. Because if our culture's deeply ingrained habits of hooking up are going to change, you and other young women, joined with young men, will be the ones to change them. Only you can shape an alternative, life-enriching vision of what relationships should look like—for one night or over a lifetime.

Do it for yourself—and for your daughters.

Gratefully yours,
Laura Sessions Stepp

Afterword to the Paperback Edition

I knew when I started to write *Unhooked,* describing the sexual landscape of young people in unsparing detail, that I would provoke reaction. What I did not foresee was how widespread the response would be—or how hungry young people are, even into their mid-twenties, to engage in honest conversations with older adults about sex and love.

Media coverage for the book was extensive. My favorite pieces were by people who applied observations in the book to their personal lives. *Cleveland Plain Dealer* columnist Connie Schultz did this; responding to a paragraph about the lack of open affection in families, she wrote about what she had seen between her parents. Her father, she recalled, used to chase her mother around the dining-room table until he caught and tickled her, and she grew up wanting *that.* She didn't achieve it in a first marriage, but has, so far, in a second, in time for her daughter, almost twenty, to catch at least a glimpse of why, as she put it, "two feet firmly planted is better than hopscotch."

Reviewers were divided. Some called the book on-target, thought-provoking and an overdue wake-up call to parents, many of whom would rather eat nails than know what was going on in the sexual lives of their high school– and college-aged children. Other reviewers— mostly women in their late thirties or early forties—were irritated by what they saw as outdated notions about sex, romance and gender roles.

Where was the harm in young women experimenting with their sexuality? they asked. Shouldn't girls be able to pursue one-night stands just like the guys? How dare I suggest how much sex women of any age should have? There was a personal edge to what some of them wrote, explained in part, perhaps, by the actively sexual pasts they admitted to.

In their reaction, they ignored the fact that *Unhooked* does not say that young women should never hook up. What I write, after reporting on teens and young adults for more than a decade, is that when young people do so repeatedly at fifteen or eighteen or twenty-one—pulling away from the love of parents and old friends, seeking new connections that comfort and inspire confidence—many get hurt, sometimes badly. *Unhooked* is simply a call for a time-out, a request that girls and adults who care about girls stop and ask some questions about what sex and relationships should look like at these tender ages.

I was not surprised that there were critics. Journalists are used to negative reactions; one can argue that we're not doing our job if we don't get at least a couple. In this case, however, the negative reviews didn't dispute my findings so much as the fact that I drew conclusions from what I had seen. They wrote as if I had spilled a dirty little secret about hooking up and in doing so, let down the team. They might expect a cautionary tale from a writer for a conservative journal, but from a *Washington Post* reporter who called herself a feminist?

The line that particularly seemed to irk a couple of these reviews came from "A Letter to Mothers and Daughters." In urging young women to get to know guys in ways other than drinking themselves under the table every weekend, I tossed out a couple of suggestions to start them thinking. Organize weekend getaways, I wrote (something one of my subjects did, with success). Or enlist other girls in baking "cookies, brownies, muffins."

"Guys will do anything for homemade baked goods," I said, remembering the delight my son took in high school and college when girls brought him chocolate chip cookies and the like. None of his girlfriends, I should note, were docile creatures—far from it. And nowhere in that section of *Unhooked*, or in any other section, was I suggesting that young women don shirtwaist dresses and frilly aprons and confine their talents to the kitchen. I was only saying that men enjoy the occasional gift, just as women do. Tickets to a basketball game would work just as well.

Readers of the age I wrote about, or close to it, understood that message and the many others in *Unhooked*. Very few of the hundreds of emails I received after publication extolled the virtues of the hookup. Instead, most of them described, sometimes in pages of detail, a personal legacy of confusion, pain and even resignation.

Their narratives arrived from all over the country and from all kinds of schools, secondary and post-secondary, public and private. Student newspapers at institutions as different as the University of Mississippi and Yale weighed in as well. According to these writers, *Unhooked* had prompted, even forced, them to step outside the social culture of which they were a part and react to what it was doing to them and/or their friends.

"I am completely lost in this hookup game," a high school senior from Chicago admitted. Another young woman, a sophomore at the University of Central Florida, wrote, "My friend told me that to get over a bad hookup I should hook up again." A junior at the University of Denver said, "I felt like I was the only one out there unsure about how I felt about the hookup culture."

A twenty-three-year-old woman said the book made her look at her past and start trying to figure out "how and why I had labored so intensely to become a stone-cold, emotionally unattached partner." She then told a chilling story of how, a couple of years earlier, she had cheated on a boyfriend by hooking up with an ex-boyfriend. As she was leaving the morning after, she said, the ex followed her to her car, looked her in the eye and said: "Hey, don't be angry with yourself. It's nothing unusual. Just think of it like doing the dishes."

"Like doing the dishes," she repeated.

The partner she described reminded me of the college man in *Unhooked* who said that the hookup culture "allows men to be bigger assholes." I don't think men want to be jerks, but the pressure on them at least to appear to be "getting some" can be intense. A number of men wrote to me saying that the hookup culture makes it difficult for a nice guy to find a loving partner. They said that independent-minded young women would rather hook up for a night or two than pursue a relationship, and that girls look for an attractive guy who will be fun to play with and easy to leave. Said one twenty-four-year-old man, "This doesn't leave much room for a guy who likes to take girls out to dinner and get to know them. (And we DO exist!)"

Another man compared the nice guy in the hookup culture to the "spare tire in your trunk." He wrote:

"The spare is usually small and ugly. . . . But when one of those regular tires goes flat and you're stranded between Los Angeles and Phoenix, boy are you glad you have that ugly little tire. So you get that tire on there, and what's the first thing you do when you get into town? Find the nearest tire place and get a normal tire put on and the ugly little spare goes back into the trunk without so much as a thank-you. . . . The good-looking asshole will get the girl every time. We are only considered as the alternate choice."

Unhooked also drew reaction from older women who remembered, none too fondly, the casual sexual encounters of their younger years. While some people have been having casual sex for decades with no noticeable impact on their emotions or their health, it wasn't true for them.

A fifty-two-year-old married woman wrote that hookups she had years ago "continue to affect my behavior and thought patterns." A forty-five-year-old single woman said she has had enough experiences to know "how damaging a lifestyle of casual sex can be." And a Marin County, California, resident, wrote: "I had a conversation with someone I went to college with in the sixties, discussing those free-loving years. He said, 'You brought a lot of pleasure to a lot of guys.' Yeah, but I got nothing out of it other than a case of VD, as I recall."

At least past generations of young women felt they had a choice whether to engage in casual sex or not. Dating was common in high school and college until a decade or so ago, and even among those who didn't date, many hoped to. Today, since hooking up has replaced dating as the social norm, young women can feel as if they have no opportunities to do anything else. They see no way out.

Listen to Courtney Tighe, a senior at Georgetown University, who wrote in her student newspaper after *Unhooked* came out:

"A man walks up to you, talks to you for seven minutes . . . and then invites you to his apartment. . . . You say, 'No thanks . . . but how about we go to the Papa Razzi sometime?' At this point you realize that you are completely alone in the room, like some kind of hideous leper. That man has just walked out the door with some other girl who wasn't so demanding."

Maybe after college, said Tighe, women will find satisfactory relationships, but it's also possible they'll end up living with ninety-two cats. It doesn't matter, she concluded: "There is no way to get out of the hookup culture . . . we can't abandon the concept that men and

women should be completely and totally equal, so there's no way to justify telling women that they can't act like men in any realm, including the
sexual one."

This is part of the conversation that older adults, in particular older
women, need to take up. Tighe's conclusion supports what I say in my
"Letter to Mothers and Daughters:" We older feminists need to elaborate on our earlier messages about equality. We need to tell them that it
isn't a question of the right to act like men. It is the opportunity to choose
whether to do that, based on what they—and not some guy or even their
best friend—know is right for them.

They need to hear that being equal doesn't have to mean being the
same. Being equal means being able, as men are able, to choose to live
and love and even lead the country in a way that is consistent with their
values. *That* is liberation.

It means continuing to work after giving birth, as presidential candidate Hillary Clinton did, or deciding to stay home with your children,
as House Speaker Nancy Pelosi did, or combining both. It can also mean
jumping a guy's bones the first time you meet or insisting on time and
opportunities to become acquainted. Both are choices. I believe the latter one is better for high school and college women, but I believe even
more strongly that they should feel free to make that choice without feeling like the odd one out. And feel free to make it again and again, no matter what they chose the last time.

Hookups are not just a matter of power. They're also a matter of
health—emotional as well as physical. This, too, needs to be part of the
conversation.

As the emails continued to arrive, virtually every day, I began to suspect
that I may have been the first adult to talk straightforwardly to my readers about the most intimate parts of their lives. Their hunger for con-

versation was palpable; a surprising number of them even asked me to write them back, which I did.

A seventeen-year-old who had read about *Unhooked* on myspace.com. wrote: "I have to be honest, at first I was very skeptical about the book. I thought, considering you did not grow up in the time or generation of the hookup culture, your opinion and ideas would be somewhat jaded. I was completely wrong. . . . I would be more than happy to talk to you."

A woman ten years older said, "I'm at a bit of a loss because I have no idea where to start finding true love. . . . Any advice?"

Not all of them were sloughing alone through the world of their feelings. A few said a parent had given *Unhooked* to them to read. Several young women said they were giving *Unhooked* to their mothers to read (not their fathers . . . hmm). In these cases connections were already in place—paying off as the children's lives became more complicated.

But many young emailers appeared to be going it alone, with little support for the internal struggles around intimacy that are so much a part of their stage in life. A forty-three-year-old mother of two teenage daughters fumed about a conversation she had had with other mothers at a Mom's Night Out.

She had told them she was concerned that her almost sixteen-year-old was not interested in boyfriends or dating. Her friends, all of whom had teenagers, said they thought this was a good thing and that girls have plenty of time for such "distractions" later.

"My response was that this is the time for them to learn how to negotiate boy-girl relationships and learn about themselves," the mother continued. "What happens if they miss this learning time and then are thrown directly into the fire in college with no supervision, no rules, no knowledge, and with expectations that are beyond their experience?"

Unhooked, she said, "has pretty well answered my questions" and she planned to use it to jump start conversations with her daughters.

The head-in-the-sand approach that she found so frightening among her friends is not because parents don't love their kids or want what's good for them. It's just that as children move into their late teens and early twenties, parents often make the mistake of thinking their daughters and sons don't want to hear what they, the gray heads, have to say. It is also the case that parents sometimes don't want to hear what their kids might tell them, and so they avoid anything approaching candor. Or, as one mother said, parents confine guidance to enrolling their children in sex education classes and getting off the occasional one-liner.

This mother wrote to tell me that she had recently come across a document in her computer that her sixteen-year-old daughter had written about performing oral sex on a guy a year earlier. As Mom read it, "my legs felt weak, my stomach grew nauseated and my world came crashing down all around me. She wrote about it all so casually."

Mother and daughter had several loud fights over the next several days about what Mom had learned. "What is wrong with you?" her daughter asked in that condescending way girls perfect during puberty. "If a boy did this, he'd be a player . . . a girl does it, she's a slut. I thought you were all for equal rights between men and women."

"I want her to hold herself in high consideration and esteem," this mother continued. "Clearly she is not there. So I continue my job as her mom. Screaming and berating got us nowhere. Understanding by way of open conversation, discussion and mutual respect (oh dear God will that be hard when she puts forth her take on sex) are in order."

Amen to that.

That mother, and several other mothers and fathers who wrote to me, sounded as painfully alone in their attempts to help their children as the children sounded describing problems with their social lives. This strengthened my conviction that today's parents cannot, by themselves, help young people navigate the shoals of sexuality safely. The best adult support, it seems to me, is a combination of parent and outside other.

As *Unhooked*'s Sienna wrote to me after she had read the whole book, her conversations with me enabled her to talk more openly to her mother, and their discussions gave her more to talk about the next time she saw me. "Though I know four years of temptation await me (at college)," she wrote, "I enter them with the wariness of experience, armed with the morals with which my parents have raised me, and the scars I suffered when I foolishly forgot their importance."

I was heartened to hear from professors, teachers, counselors and church youth workers who are pitching in. A drama coach wrote about her new job at the University of Minnesota. She said she had been shocked at the explicitness of a play the students had been assigned before she arrived, and nonplussed at the students' own blasé attitudes about its raw and violent sexuality. She was no prude, she assured me. "Having been a late seventies/early eighties teen and twentysomething . . . I had a lot of fun in college 'finding myself.' But recently I've realized how far away I am from what is happening with the young women I'm teaching now."

She had decided she couldn't ignore what she was seeing. "There is art," she wrote, "and then there is pornography. I wonder if the lines are blurred for them. I hope I can help them see the difference, which is relationship. *Othello* is a tragedy because of the depth of [Othello's] love, not merely the depth of his sexual jealousy. That's what keeps it from being a TV movie."

A youth minister at a small church in Texas admitted that before reading *Unhooked,* her advice to a college prep class each summer was not to take relationships too seriously. This was based on her own experiences, she said, "of falling too hard too fast for someone and the emotional turmoil that accompanies a relationship like that. . . . I now see how that can communicate a condonement of the hookup culture. I'll be reevaluating the advice I offer and center around respect for the other person and what committed love can bring to the relationship."

A health professor at George Washington University wrote saying he had introduced the subject of hooking up into his standard lectures about sexually transmitted diseases. A teacher at a private secondary school in McLean, Virginia, assigned passages from *Unhooked* to her psychology students and asked them to write about their reactions. She then invited me to come speak to the classes.

Near the end of one class, several senior girls told me they wanted to start a dating club at school. We joked that they should have T-shirts printed that read, "Ask me for a date."

Did I think a club like that would work? the girls asked. What else could they do to inject romance into their social lives?

Their questions, like so many responses I was receiving, convinced me that young people not only want us to listen to their ideas about sex and love, they want to know what we think.

Sometimes, however, we must choose our words carefully.

A college junior wrote that she had spent two years in the hookup culture at her school and was in the process of trying to extricate herself from it. She was hoping to find someone to love, and a conversation with her grandmother had not been particularly encouraging.

"Is there anyone special in your life right now?" Grandma had asked.

"When I told her 'No,' her response was, 'Good,' " the young woman wrote. "I said, 'Excuse me?' and she said that she wouldn't want falling in love to get in the way of me completing my degree."

The young woman continued, "I am a motivated individual [who] would NEVER drop out of my almost $200,000 investment for any guy." But it would have been nice to get a little encouragement for her dream, she said.

Our conversations must value young people's dual needs for independence *and* a deeply satisfying, intimate life. This was why I wrote the last chapter, "A Letter to Mothers and Daughters," explaining how I thought young women could have both.

I had done so after some hesitation, for I did not want young readers to think that, after laying out the hookup scene in careful, objective detail, I was slamming them for taking part in it. Emails I received after publication told me my readers did not feel that way; on the contrary, they felt reassured.

A college sophomore wrote, "I want to copy your letter and paste it to every wall in my apartment, to have it around me." A college graduate on her way to medical school said:

"I cannot read the chapter 'A Letter to Mothers and Daughters' without crying. I am valuable, I am the subject of my own life, my body is my own property, I am classy, hooking up is never meaningless, drinking is not an excuse and I will not be used. Thank you for reminding me of all these things. . . . I will pass the message along!"

Such responses remind us that the goal of adult intervention is not to tell young people what to do—as if we could. It is to encourage introspection and give them, where needed, the courage either to change what they do according to what they know deep down they want, or continue to do what is making them feel healthy and strong. Some of the most satisfying emails I received told stories about girls who had found such encouragement in *Unhooked*.

"This past weekend I was at a party where I found myself talking with a guy friend I had hooked up with the previous semester," wrote a student at a Pennsylvania college who had just finished the book. "We started making out and by the time we had reached my bedroom, I had gone through a complete thought process and was able to reject him, without feeling bad and actually feeling empowered by my ability to say no. Kudos to the young women who shared their stories, their heartbreak and their life lessons. I for one am extremely grateful."

A nineteen-year-old woman from Southern Maryland wrote that she was starting a discussion group with other young women to talk about relationships and life choices. A 2004 graduate of Columbia University wrote to say that she had made a feature-length film about her experiences in a "hypersexualized college with no one to guide me and no one stable to rely on." After reading *Unhooked*, she said, she better understood what she went through in college and what motivated her to make the film, which she hoped would spur conversation on current sexual trends.

These are smart young women who, like many of their generation, are in the process of realizing that what goes on between two brains is just as important as what goes on between two bodies, and that the combination of brains and bodies is powerful indeed. It was great to hear from some who had already discovered that.

One, a twenty-one-year-old senior at Tulane University in New Orleans, wrote that she hooked up on and off during her college years until she met a young man, twenty-six, near the end of first semester senior year. They dated for a couple of months until he moved to San Francisco to take a new job. "Smart, handsome, funny, good-hearted—he was everything I always wanted," she said.

She still goes to bars with her girlfriends, she continued, but has been celibate since he left because she hasn't met anyone who could compare to him. She has applied to graduate schools all over the country, including one in San Francisco. But, she wrote, she's actually hoping to get into an East Coast school, and is "sure" there is another man out there for her like her former boyfriend.

She discovered, as Alicia in *Unhooked* discovered, that being in love, or at least being in a relationship even if you're reluctant to call it love, can make anything else seem second-rate. So did a college junior who wrote that she had made "some serious changes in my behavior when it comes to guys and hooking up. I still go out to parties or bars with my girlfriends on occasion," she said, "but I'm no longer on the prowl. If a guy approaches me, there's no way I'm making out in a dark corner of a club or consider going home with him. I am very proud of myself for figuring out what is healthy for me.

"Although I had already made a lot of progress on my own toward dragging myself out of the hookup culture, your book gave me encouragement to keep up my efforts. . . . I guess I'll just have to keep waiting until I find that man who opens doors, brings me flowers for no reason, kisses me on the forehead and encourages all my aspirations."

As my husband recently reminded me, *Unhooked* is not really about having less sex. It's about having more love—as annoying, foolish, and impractical as love can be.

Acknowledgments

Unhooked grew out of articles about the sexual habits of adolescents and young adults that I wrote over several years at *The Washington Post*. Many newspaper editors would rather swallow toads than publish such accounts, and I am lucky indeed that my editors at the paper are not in that group. Beginning with executive editor Len Downie, they grasped the importance of the subject, gave me the time to pursue it, and displayed my stories appropriately.

Special thanks go to Style editors Gene Robinson, Deborah Heard and Steve Reiss for their support. My immediate editor, Henry Allen, is simply the best, and continues to inspire me as a reporter, writer and thinker. Other colleagues in the *Post*'s Style section acted as both sounding boards and hand-holders; they include Libby Copeland, Ann Corbett, Jennifer Frey and Joel Garreau. I am especially indebted to Ann Gerhart for her ideas, Alison Howard for her editing and William Raspberry for his wisdom and unfailing sense of humor.

A reporter is only as good as her sources. To my primary sources—

the young women and their families—I owe enormous thanks for their candor and courage. Thanks also to those who work for the universities I write about—in particular Donna Lisker, Larry Moneta and Susan Roth at Duke University; and Mark Feldstein, Heather Schell and Mary Jo Warner at George Washington University. The early support of GW president Stephen Joel Trachtenberg and former Duke president Keith Brodie also meant a great deal.

Several experts helped me place the experiences of the young women of *Unhooked* within the adolescent/young adult culture at large. They include William Beardslee, professor of child psychiatry, Harvard University; Robert Blum, chair, Bloomberg School of Public Health, Johns Hopkins University; Jane Brown, professor of journalism and mass communication, University of North Carolina–Chapel Hill; Rosemary Chalk, director, Board on Children, Youth and Families, Institute of Medicine and National Research Council; Kathleen Mullen Harris, professor of sociology, University of North Carolina–Chapel Hill; Lloyd Kolbe, professor of health education, Indiana University–Bloomington; Jennifer Manlove, director, Suzanne Ryan, senior research associate and Kerry Franzetta, research analyst, Child Trends; Laurence Steinberg, professor of psychology, Temple University; and Richard Udry, professor of sociology, University of North Carolina–Chapel Hill.

Sarah Brown, executive director of the National Campaign to Prevent Teen Pregnancy, along with the Campaign's Bill Albert and Marisa Nightingale, provided invaluable advice and support from beginning to end. Several other organizations, embracing a range of points of view, were also helpful, among them Advocates for Youth, the Boys & Girls Club of America and the National Marriage Project at Rutgers University.

It is possible I might not ever have started writing *Unhooked* had it not been for the early and relentless encouragement of three people: crime novelist Patricia Cornwell; health journalist Cheree Cleghorn; and Tom

Kunkel, dean of the College of Journalism at the University of Maryland and, more important, father of four daughters. Other friends who sustained me are Arnold and Judy Baker, Jerry and Carol Barney, Cindy Farber-Soule, Beth Frerking and David Wood, Gail Gomila, Don and Marcy Leverenz, Elena Nightingale, Al and Alfie Rulis and Deborah Yaeger.

I cannot possibly thank all the young people who were willing to consider my ideas and tell me when I was right and, more important, when I was off base. Among those I must mention are the terrific students I taught at George Washington University: Brian Calvary, Sacha Evans, Tony Moniello, Christy Samuels, Jessica Smith, Andrew White and Emily Zeigenfuse. Three other students in that class—Mariam Alkazemi, Sarah Belanger and Sarah Halzak—assisted in outside research as well. In addition, I would like to thank Liz Finch and friends of Duck, North Carolina; Jennifer and Kimberly Kramer of Bethesda, Maryland; Emily Mauro of Alexandria, Virginia; Thea Soule of Rochester, New York; and Paige Plissner, Nick Kaplan and Ashley Wilson of Washington, D.C.

My gratitude to the W. T. Grant Foundation for underwriting the data analysis by Child Trends, and to Susan Dales and the Frameworks Institute for facilitating the grant process and supporting my work. I was the lucky recipient of a Shapiro Fellowship at GW and thank, in particular, Mark Feldstein and Steven Livingston for making that possible. Thanks also to Michele Masset for her support when *Unhooked* was a germ of an idea, and to publisher/editor Charles Cornwell for his insights as the writing of the book came to a close.

Thank you, Esther Newberg, for your vision, as my agent, of what is possible, and for helping make the possible real. Thanks to Cindy Spiegel, Riverhead's former copublisher, for seeing the book's potential, and to my editor, Jake Morrissey, for his ideas, patience and ability to make me laugh when I most needed it. I count myself lucky to be with Riverhead Books again.

I was delighted to be invited once more to serve as a visiting scholar at the Board on Children, Youth and Families, a collaborative effort of the Institute of Medicine and the National Research Council. My thanks to Christine Hartel, director of the Center for Studies of Behavior and Development, and to Rosemary Chalk, for making the appointment happen and giving me an office in which I could work. I had many useful conversations with Board staff and would like to thank specifically Wendy Keenan, Jessica Martinez and Donna Randall.

When I needed solitude, I traveled to one of my favorite places in the world, North Carolina's Outer Banks, where I stayed in homes owned by my friends Georgia and Olin Finch. Thanks to them both for the ocean views and our conversations.

I am fortunate to have a patient family, in particular my parents, sisters, grown children and saint of a husband, who provided a sharp editor's eye and regular dinners. A final note to my son Jeff, now working in Los Angeles, who put up with a mother who, throughout his adolescence, wrote articles that sometimes embarrassed him. Thank you, Jeff, for encouraging me to do such stories anyway—and for helping me understand that despite occasional appearances to the contrary, young people simply want what the rest of us want, to love and be loved.

Notes

Section One. Hooking Up: What It Means

page 33   *"Everyone here seems intent": Morning Edition*, National Public Radio, November 20, 1996.

page 33   *A year later, in 1997:* Trip Gabriel, "Campus Courting More Casual," *The New York Times*, January 27, 1997.

page 33   *A major research project:* The Women's Initiative of Duke University assessed the situation of women among various Duke constituencies: undergraduates, graduate and professional students, alumnae, faculty, employees and board of trustees. The report, known as "Duke Inquiries in Gender," is referred to several times throughout this book, usually as the Duke study.

page 33   *In 2000, Elizabeth Paul:* Daniel McGinn, "Mating Behavior 101," *Newsweek*, October 4, 2004.

page 34   *Accounts in the late 1990s of hooking up:* Laura Sessions Stepp, "Parents Are Alarmed by an Unsettling New Fad in Middle Schools: Oral Sex," *The Washington Post*, July 8, 1999. Parents may also be interested in a sidebar to that article that ran on the same day, titled "Talking to Kids about Sexual Limits."

page 34   *Researchers at Bowling Green State University:* Laura Sessions Stepp, "The Buddy System; Sex in High School and College: What's Love Got to Do with It?," *The Washington Post*, January 19, 2003.

page 34   *In mid-2005, a study funded:* The CDC study is titled "Sexual Behavior and Selected Health Measures: Men and Women 15–44 Years of Age, United States, 2002." It was published in September 2005. For the purposes of this book, Child Trends, a nonprofit, nonpartisan research organization in Washington, D.C., analyzed data contained in this study, as well as data from two other national sources: The National Longitudinal Study of Adolescent Health and the National Longitudinal Survey of Youth. You may find out more about Child Trends at www.childtrends.org.

page 36   *In her book* From Front Porch to Back Seat*:* Beth L. Bailey, *From Front Porch to Back Seat: Courtship in Twentieth-Century America* (Baltimore: Johns Hopkins University Press, 1989), pp. 23–24. This is an excellent resource on the history of courtship in the United States, particularly among the middle class, during the first three-quarters of the century.

page 36   *For about ten years, beginning in the early 1920s:* Gail Collins, *America's Women: 400 Years of Dolls, Drudges, Helpmates and Heroines* (New York: Perennial/HarperCollins, 2003), pp. 328–30. For an entertaining and insightful look at a clash of two generations, young and old, which resembles ours today, read the entire chapter.

page 37   *Statistics confound the once common assumption:* Child Trends reports, 2003–2005.

page 38   *Columnists opined at length about:* Centers for Disease Control and Prevention, "Sexual Behavior and Selected Health Measures, 2002," p. 34.

page 39   *Females' sexual assertiveness mirrors:* For the most current figures regarding women's educational status, see the website of the National Center for Education Statistics, at nces.ed.gov. One useful report is titled "Trends in Educational Equity of Girls & Women."

page 39   *When Congress, in 1972, passed Title IX:* Bill Pennington, "Title IX Trickles Down to Girls of Generation Z," *The New York Times,* June 29, 2004.

page 48   *Researchers estimate that before reaching college:* Jeffrey Jensen Arnett, *Adolescence and Emerging Adulthood* (Upper Saddle River, N.J.: Pearson/Prentice Hall, 2004), p. 386.

page 48   *A 2005 study revealed:* Kaiser Family Foundation, "Sex on TV 4," report released November 9, 2005.

page 50   *Ninety percent of adolescents:* Arnett, *Adolescence and Emerging Adulthood,* p. 407.

page 50   *More than half of older adolescents:* John Consoli, "Teen Cell Subs Heavy TV Users," May 3, 2005, www.mediaweek.com. Also see Arnett, *Adolescence and Emerging Adulthood,* p. 409.

page 53   Stories of love, both mythological: Helen Fisher, *Why We Love: The Nature and Chemistry of Romantic Love* (New York: Henry Holt, 2004), p. 3.

page 53   In the nineteenth and early twentieth centuries: Lewis Carroll, *Letters of a Nation* (New York: Broadway, 1999).

page 53   But by the 1930s, scientists: Peter Stearns and Mark Knapp, "Men and Romantic Love: Pinpointing a 20th-Century Change," *Journal of Social History*, Summer 1993.

Section Two. What It Looks Like, What It Feels Like

page 75   According to national data released in mid-2005: Centers for Disease Control and Prevention, "Sexual Behavior and Selected Health Measures, 2002," p. 25; and analysis by Child Trends.

page 79   In one eighteen-month study, James Moody: Peter S. Bearman, James Moody and Katharine Stovel, "Chains of Affection," *American Journal of Sociology*, July 2004.

page 101   Jonetta Rose Barras wrote: Jonetta Rose Barras, *Whatever Happened to Daddy's Little Girl? The Impact of Fatherlessness on Black Women* (New York: One World/Ballantine, 2002).

page 102   Indeed, national studies show: Analysis by Child Trends.

page 118   The feeling of lust: For a discussion of the difference between lust, romance and attachment, see Fisher, *Why We Love*, pp. 77–98.

page 123   Moderate drinking among college-aged students: National Institutes of Health, U.S. Department of Health & Human Services, "Monitoring the Future, 2003 (Trends in Alcohol and Cigarette Use: College Students)." Also see www.hsph.harvard.edu/cas/.

page 123   Young women who play such games: Thomas J. Johnson, "Sexual Experiences Associated with Participation in Drinking Games," *Journal of General Psychology*, July 2004.

page 125   According to Leslie Campis: Statistics in this paragraph come from a presentation by Campis to the Department of Psychiatry, Children's Hospital, Boston, June 2006.

page 132   In certain stressful situations: S. E. Taylor et al., "Biobehavioral responses to stress in females: Tend-and-befriend, not fight-or-flight," *Psychological Review*, 107 (2000), pp. 411–29.

page 137   Barbara Dafoe Whitehead: David Popenoe and Barbara Dafoe Whitehead, *The State of Our Unions, 2000 Special Report: Sex Without Strings, Rela-*

tionships Without Rings: Today's Young Singles Talk About Mating and Dating (New Brunswick: National Marriage Project, Rutgers University, June 2000).

page 138   *Anthropologist Fisher discovered:* Fisher, *Why We Love*, pp. 51–76.

Section Three. How We Got There

page 155   *Lynn Harris, a writer in her twenties:* Lynn Harris, "I'm Norah Jonesing," *Glamour*, September 2004, p. 168.

page 158   *Not much difference between:* These letters and others referenced later in this chapter appeared in *The Chronicle*, Duke's student newspaper, on various dates in late 2004 and early 2005.

page 159   *Married Muslim women are:* Paula Drew, "Iran," *The International Encyclopedia of Sexuality*, ed. by Robert T. Francoeur (New York: Continuum, 1997–2001).

page 183   *This generation of kids:* Barry Schwarz, "The Tyranny of Choice," *Scientific American*, April 2004.

page 183   *National surveys have documented:* Two well-researched studies of time use are: F. Thomas Juster et al., "Changing Times of American Youth, 1981–2003" (Ann Arbor: Institute for Social Research, University of Michigan, November 2004) and "All Work and No Play?" (released in November 2004 by Public Agenda, a nonpartisan research organization in Washington, D.C.; available at http://www.publicagenda.org/research/pdfs/all_work_no_ play.pdf).

page 184   *The stress-for-success that can result:* Amanda Paulson, *The Christian Science Monitor*, March 21, 2005.

page 184   *"Taking on only one thing":* Whitney Beckett, "Rights on an Exclusive," *The Chronicle*, November 14, 2003.

page 191   *Several years ago, social commentator Kay Hymowitz:* Kay S. Hymowitz, *Liberation's Children: Parents and Kids in a Postmodern Age* (Chicago: Ivan Dee, 2003), pp. 124–25.

page 193   *The AARP in 2003:* Xenia Montenegro, "Lifestyles, Dating and Romance: A Study of Midlife Singles" (Washington, D.C.: AARP, September 2003).

page 196   *According to those who study generational differences:* Neil Howe and William Strauss, *Millennials Rising: The Next Great Generation* (New York: Vintage, 2000), pp. 12–24.

page 198   "At Harvard, we know competition": Angie Marek, "What Is Cheating?" *The Harvard Crimson*, December 5, 2002.

page 204   "At Duke, we're on a fast-paced track": Anne Katharine Wales, "Holding on to Dreams," *The Chronicle*, December 1, 2004.

page 213   *When this country was founded:* Nancy L. Thomas, "The New In Loco Parentis," *Change* 23 (September/October 1991), pp. 32–40. Thomas, an education law specialist, summarizes the history of college regulations and argues for better education of students rather than more rules.

page 213   "Every possible aspect of student life": Cited in Thomas, "The New In Loco Parentis."

page 214   *As Wendy White:* Wendy S. White, "Students, Parents, Colleges: Drawing the Lines," *The Chronicle of Higher Education*, December 16, 2005.

page 216   *In the late 1980s, several colleges:* Thomas, "The New In Loco Parentis." Also see David A. Hoekma, "College Life in America: Historical Context and Legal Issues," in *New Directions for Student Services* (Hoboken, N.J.: Jossey-Bass, 1996), pp. 3–17.

page 217   *Not all educators agree:* Vigen Guroian, "Dorm Brothel," *Christianity Today*, February 2005, p. 23.

page 220   *Increasing opportunities for such discussion:* Vu Le, "We Need a Class on Romantic Relationships," *Student Life*, May 3, 2004.

page 222   *As Marline Pearson, a college teacher:* Marline Pearson, Speech at Smart Marriages Conference, Reno, Nevada, June 2003; found at http://marriage.rutgers.edu.

page 223   *Generational experts Neil Howe and William Strauss:* Howe and Strauss, *Millennials*, pp. 52, 109–10.

page 231   *Well over half of college students:* Donna Freitas, "Excess and Longing," *The Wall Street Journal*, May 20, 2005. Also see Laura Sessions Stepp, "An Inspired Strategy: Is Religion a Tonic for Kids?" *The Washington Post*, March 21, 2004.

Section Four. Hooking Up: Why It Matters

page 237   *In a survey of 1,000 college women:* Noval D. Glenn and Elizabeth Marquardt, "Hooking Up, Hanging Out and Hoping for Mr. Right: College Women on Dating and Mating Today," Institute for American Values, July 26, 2001, p. 16.

page 238   *The pregnancy rate among girls:* The statistics on this and the following
           page are drawn from the CDC study "Sexual Behavior and Selected
           Health Measures, 2002," as well as the National Campaign to Prevent
           Teen Pregnancy (rates of pregnancy and abortion); Guttmacher Institute
           and Contraception Online, Baylor College of Medicine (rates of STDs);
           and Myra G. Schneider et al., "Association of Psychosocial Factors with
           the Stress of Infertility Treatment," *Health and Social Work*, August 1, 2005
           (infertility).

page 241   *Girls, more than guys, report:* Deborah P. Welsh et al., "When Love Hurts:
           Depression and Adolescent Romantic Relationships," in Paul Florsheim,
           ed., *Adolescent Romantic Relations and Sexual Behavior* (Mahwah, N.J.:
           Lawrence Erlbaum Associates, 2003), pp. 200–201. Also see "Adolescent
           Lovers Studied" (February 14, 2001), a summary of a study by sociologists
           Kara Joyner of Cornell University and J. Richard Udry of the University
           of North Carolina–Chapel Hill, found at www.hypography.com.

page 242   *Young women may be at greatest risk:* Richard Kadison, *College of the Over-
           whelmed* (Hoboken, N.J.: Jossey-Bass, 2004), pp. 95–96. Also, data from the
           National College Health Assessment (American College Health Associa-
           tion), Spring 2005; and presentation by Bradford D. King, director, Student
           Counseling Services, University of Southern California, at annual meet-
           ing of the Society for Adolescent Medicine, March 30, 2005.

page 244   *In the United States, anorexia:* Kadison, pp. 131–33. Also see website of
           the National Association of Anorexia Nervosa & Related Disorders,
           www.anad.org.

page 248   *Faculty sponsors of the Duke report on gender:* "Duke Inquiries in Gender,"
           p. 3.

page 252   *One out of five girls in college:* "Sexual Assault on Campus . . . ," p. 2.

page 262   *These young people have grown up in a country:* Andrew Cherlin, "American
           Marriage in the Early Twenty-first Century," *Marriage and Child Wellbe-
           ing* 15 (Fall 2005), p. 46, and Karen S. Peterson, "Divorce Need Not End
           in Disaster," *USA Today*, January 13, 2002.

page 264   *And let's not forget that a large number:* Laura Sessions Stepp, "In Spring, a
           Young Man's Fancy Turns to Work," *The Washington Post*, March 26, 2006.

page 265   *In the last part of the nineteenth century:* Collins, *America's Women*, p. 294.

page 265   *Beginning in the 1960s:* Steven Bodzin, "Home Alone: Households of Sin-
           gles Go to First in U.S.," *Los Angeles Times*, August 18, 2005.

Index

Education on sexual topics, 221–22
Einstein, Albert, 53
Electronic media, adolescents and, 50–51
Emily (GW junior), 219
Emotions, hooking up and, 27, 237
Empowerment of women, 152–53
Ensler, Eve, *The Vagina Monologues,* 166–72, 228
Erotic sex, 282–83
Esquire magazine, 53
Ethnic differences in sexual activity, 102

Faculty members, and campus life, 213
Family honor, 72
Fathers
    and daughters, 45–46
    lack of emotional support from, 100, 101, 165
    relationships with, 107–8, 225–26
Female friendships, 130–34
Feminism, 16, 37, 38, 292
    and dating system, 36
    and expectations, 182
    and relationships, 234
    and unhooked culture, 151–79
Fisher, Helen, *Why We Love,* 118–19, 138
Flapper generation, 36–37
Flirtation, 36, 284
    feminist view, 154
Fraternities, 215
    Duke University, 21, 24–25
    George Washington University, 116
"Free love," 28, 154
Free to Be You and Me, Thomas, 197
Freedom
    of college life, 113
    sexual, 36–37
Freitas, Donna, 232
French, Marilyn, *The Women's Room,* 191
French, Sandy, 92
Freud, Sigmund, 187
Frey, Bill, 267
Friedan, Betty, 154
Friends, influence of, 50
Friendships, 15, 130–34, 281–82
From Front Porch to Back Seat, Bailey, 36
Future, consideration of, 277

Gay population, female, 13–14
Gender equality, 36–38, 159, 292
    in classrooms, 39
Gender roles, in relationships, 81–82
Generational changes in behavior, 2, 4–5
Genital herpes, 239
George Washington University (GW), 13, 113–14, 295–96
    "date auction," 3–4
Girls, use of term, 12
    See also Women
Gladwell, Malcolm, *The Tipping Point,* 44
Goals, set by parents, 194
Government, federal, and sexuality studies, 33–34
Grades, hooking up and, 80
Gray rape, 248–49
    See also Sexual assault
Greek organizations (fraternities, sororities)
    and alcohol, 126
    Duke University, 21, 24–25
Groups, adolescent, behavior defined by, 72–74, 79
Guroian, Vigen, 217
GW. *See* George Washington University

Haitian immigrants, 208, 224–25
Harris, Camille, 97–98
Harris, Lynn, 155
Harvard College, early days, 213
Harvard Crimson, The, and cheating, 198
Harvard School of Public Health, alcohol study, 123
Hawthorne, Nathaniel, 53
Head-in-the-sand approach to hookup culture, 293–94
Health counseling services, 221
Hell with Love, The, 137
High school students, 65
    all-girl schools, 115, 182
    private school, 67–84
    public school, 84–96
    and religion, 231
    sexual activity, 37–38
        hooking up, 34–35, 145
HIV infections, 238–39
Holding hands in public, 260
Hooking up, xiv, 5, 15, 17, 144–45, 236, 282
    alcohol and, 123–25, 289
    Alicia's view, 270–71

fear of, 203
feminism and, 154, 191–92
Jamie's story, 54–64
and lust, 118–19
of self, 277–79
sex and, 7
young women and, 15
Lust, 118–19, 280

Magazines, 50
Male behavior, young women and, 65–66
Maria (friend of Anna), 95
Marić, Mileva, 53
Marie (mother of Victoria), 208, 224–28
Mark (Sienna's hookup partner), 79–82
Marriage
age of, 263
attitudes to, 9, 22, 24, 41–42, 226
parents' relationships and, 42–43, 52
cheating and, 257
failures of, 262
good, qualities of, 252–53
hooking up and, 238
views of, 187, 191–93, 233
feminist, 154
Maximizers, 183–84
Media, and sexual behavior, 47–51
Medical schools, female enrollment, 39
Memories, 280–81
Men, 6, 272–73
and dating, 35–37
and hooking up, 38, 290
Michael (Nicole's boyfriend), 134–35, 136–37,
139–44, 145–46
Middle schools, hooking up in, 34
Middle-school students, oral sex, 1–2
Mieka (public high school student), 15, 96–110,
144, 165, 258
Minorities, immigrant, 208
Moderation in behavior, students and, 73
Monika (Mieka's friend), 98–99, 104, 110
Monogamy, 207–8
Moody, James, 79
Moore, Alice Ruth, 53
Morgan (GW freshman), 3–4, 125–26
Motherhood, careers and, 265
Mothers
and daughters, 44–46, 144

marriage relationships, 42–43
unmarried, 265, 266
Multitasking, 184
Muslim women, 159
My Freshman Year, 273
myspace.com, 293

Nasim (mother of Shaida), 156, 157–59, 165–66
and *The Vagina Monologues,* 171–72
Nate (Nicole's hookup partner), 129, 146
Nathan (Shaida's hookup partner), 175–77
National Campaign to Prevent Teen Pregnancy,
10, 267
Necking, 37
Nicholas (Victoria's boyfriend), 208, 210–11,
230–31
Nicole (GW sophomore, Cleo's sister), 15, 16, 46,
48, 111–47, 162, 182, 255–56
Cleo and, 187–88
Nightingale, Marisa, 267
Niko (father of Cleo and Nicole), 114, 136, 189,
190
Noah (Anna's crush), 92–93, 94
Nolen-Hoeksema, Susan, 241

Objectives set by parents, 194
OC, The (TV show), 49–50
O'Connell, Mark, 32
Older men, sex with, 102
Older women, friendship with, 282
One-night stands, 74–75
Online dating services, 264
Open relationships, 206
Opportunities for women, feminism and, 182
Oral sex, 74, 75, 90–91, 92, 168
CDC report, 38
and disease, 239
in high school, 69
middle-school students and, 1–2
Our Last Best Shot, Stepp, 8
Oxytocin, intercourse and, 129–30

Parents, xv, 5, 10–11, 14, 16, 17, 44–46, 83
and alcohol consumption, 124
and attitudes to love, 52
and culture, 149, 273
unhooked culture, 180–206
divorced, 85, 262

and freedom of campus life, 214–15
and high school students, 71–73
and hooking up, 40–42, 144–45, 293–95
investment in daughters, 182
Jamie and, 23–24
relationship between, 42–43, 225–26, 266
conflict, 165–66
love, 136
unmarried, 97, 107–8
Parties, high school students and, 77–79, 87
Partners, exchange of, 78
Patty (Nicole's friend), 113, 119, 121–23, 127–28, 129–34, 137, 141
Paul, Elizabeth, 33
Payne, Mary Louise, 88
Payne, Robert, 88
Peabody, Sophia, 53
Pearson, Marline, 222
Peer approval, and sexual behavior, 72–74, 79
hooking up, 44, 219–20
Pelosi, Nancy, 292
Perfectionism, 69–70, 185–87, 233
Personal fulfillment, feminism and, 182
Personal responsibility, 196
Petting, 37
Physical closeness, and emotions, 240–41
Physical safety, colleges and, 222–23
"Players," girls as, 67
Pleasure, sexual, 168–69, 259
Popenoe, David, 137
Pornographic sex, 282–83
Power
feelings of, sex and, 112
wise use of, 283–84
Pregnancy, hooking up and, 238
Pressures on young women, 69–70
Private school students, 71–79
Professional success, feminism and, 182
Professors, and campus life, 213
Promiscuities, Wolf, 153
Public high schools, 79, 86–97

Rape, 176–77, 246–52
See also Sexual assault
Reactions to *Unhooked,* 287–99
"Reasonable care," colleges and, 222
Regulations, lacking in college, 213–15
Relationships, 187, 233–34, 240–43, 261–63

Alicia's view, 271
attitudes to, 4–6, 40–45, 96–98, 98–99
avoidance, 51–52
feminist, 191–92
on college campus, 54–55, 56
communications and, 76
control in, 57–64, 65
education for, 222
ending of, 51
friendships among girls, 130–34
gender roles, 81–82
in high school, 69–70
hooking up and, 5–7, 15, 27–28, 65–66, 96
intimacy in, 277
loving, 279–80
romantic, 51–54, 106
and interpersonal skills, 257
sex and, 32–33
sexual, types of, 74–75
Religion, college students and, 231–33
Research for this book, 8–14
Respect for self, 278–79
Restrictions
freedom from, in college, 212–14
parental, on daughters, 194–95
Revenge, 111–12
Reversal of gender roles, 81–82
Ringold, Jill, 216, 221
Roffman, Deborah, 10
Roiphe, Katie, 213
Role models, parents as, 16, 17
Romance, attitudes to, 15, 100–101, 106
Romantic love, 51–54
Room of One's Own, A, Woolf, 182
Rudolph, Frederick, 213

Sawyer, Robin, 32, 273–74
Schell, Heather, 137
Schools, and cultural change, 273
Schultz, Connie, 287
Scientists, and love, 53
Self, love of, 277–79
Self-confidence, development of, 277–78
Self-doubt, feelings of, 88–89
Self-esteem, sexuality and, 162
Self-sufficiency, parents and, 181
Self-worth, poor sense of, hooking up and, 251